The Acid-Alkaline Lifestyle

OTHER WORKS BY LARRY TRIVIERI, JR.

From Square One Publishers

The Acid-Alkaline Food Guide
(with Susan Brown, PhD)

Juice Alive: The Ultimate Guide to Juicing Remedies
(with Steven Bailey, ND)

Other Select Titles

Alternative Medicine: The Definitive Guide
(editor and co-writer, with Burton Goldberg)

*The American Holistic Medical Association
Guide to Holistic Health*

Chronic Fatigue, Fibromyalgia & Lyme Disease
(with Burton Goldberg)

The Complete Self-Care Guide to Holistic Medicine
(with Rob Ivker, MD and Robert Anderson, MD)

*Health On The Edge: Visionary Views of Healing
in the New Millennium*

The Acid- Alkaline Lifestyle

The Complete Program for Better Health and Vitality

LARRY TRIVIERI, JR
NEIL RAFF, MD

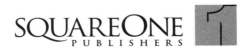

SQUAREONE
PUBLISHERS

COVER DESIGNER: Jeannie Tudor
EDITOR: Erica Shur
TYPESETTER: Gary A. Rosenberg

The information and advice contained in this book are based upon the research and the personal and professional experiences of the author. They are not intended as a substitute for consulting with a health care professional. The publisher and author are not responsible for any adverse effects or consequences resulting from the use of any of the suggestions, preparations, or procedures discussed in this book. All matters pertaining to your physical health should be supervised by a health care professional. It is a sign of wisdom, not cowardice, to seek a second or third opinion.

Square One Publishers
115 Herricks Road
Garden City Park, NY 11040
(516) 535-2010 • (877) 900-BOOK
www.squareonepublishers.com

Library of Congress Cataloging-in-Publication Data
Trivieri, Larry.
  The acid-alkaline lifestyle : the complete program for better health and vitality / Larry Trivieri Jr., Neil Raff, MD.
      pages cm
    Includes index.
  ISBN 978-0-7570-0389-9
    1. Acid-base equilibrium—Health aspects. 2. Acid-base imbalances—Diet therapy. 3. Acid-base imbalances—Nutritional aspects. 4. Self-care, Health. 5. Health. I. Raff, Neil. II. Title.
    RC630.T74   2015
    616.3'992—dc23

                                                                2014044503

Printed in the United States of America

10   9   8   7   6   5   4   3   2   1

Contents

To Bob Cohen and Richard Stark for their many years
of friendship, support, creativity, and inspiration.

To my mother, Margaret Moyer Trivieri, who first
recognized and nurtured my talents as a writer,
and whose other gifts to me are so numerous
it would take another book to list them all.

To the memory of my dear friends, Karen Defuria
Marshall and Steve Lazarek, and of my
beloved sister and niece, Andrea and Krystle.
"Some wounds aren't meant to heal."

And, most especially, to my father, Lawrence A.
Trivieri, who unexpectedly passed away while this
book was in production. Everything I am today I owe
to the example he set for me throughout his long and
well-lived life. Words cannot express the gratitude
I have for the countless blessings I received as his son.

—L.T.

To my dear wife Anne, the ultimate environmentalist,
who has created a loving, meaningful, and
supportive world for me to thrive in.

To my three sons, Dr. Harry Raff, Dr. Adam Raff,
and Dr. Joshua Raff, who provide me with unbound
joy and pride, and keep me young trying to
keep up with their accomplishments.

—N. R.

Acknowledgments

I wish to thank my friend and publisher, Rudy Shur, for his ongoing support and thoughtful suggestions. It was Rudy who first suggested to me that I create a book about the pH properties of foods and beverages. His doing so led to my writing *The Acid-Alkaline Food Guide* with Dr. Susan Brown, the success of which has led to me writing this book, as well. I would also like to thank Rudy's entire team at Square One, especially Anthony Pomes, for his marketing acumen, and Erica Shur, for her astute comments and light hand as she edited the manuscript. I also wish to thank Neil Raff for agreeing to be a part of this project and for being such an enjoyable collaborator.

I also want to acknowledge and thank my dear friend, Burton Goldberg, the only mentor I've ever had and the only one I've ever needed. More than twenty years ago, Burton saw something in me that I had yet to recognize in myself. In doing so, he opened the door to my career, and I shall never forget the powerful, positive impact he had on me when he told me one day, "Don't tell me how you fail. Tell me how you succeed!" Much gratitude and love, old friend!

My thanks, as well, to the many brilliant and dedicated physicians and other health experts it has been my good fortune to know and learn from, with a special tip of my cap to Drs. C. Norman Shealy, Garry Gordon, Michael Galitzer, Alan Gaby, Kenneth

Singleton, Robert Ivker, Robert A. Anderson, Rashid Buttar, Susan Brown, and the late, great Valerie Hunt.

Finally, and most importantly, I once again want to acknowledge my family and friends, both of which are large tribes that is my very great fortune to be loved and supported by. My deepest thanks to every single one of them for all that we continue to share.

—Larry Trivieri Jr

I would like to acknowledge the three doctors who greatly influenced my training and thinking. Phillip Tumulty, MD, Professor of Medicine at Johns Hopkins School of Medicine, as brilliant and all-knowing as he was, always emphasized caring for the patients and their needs, not the patients and their diagnosis. Adam Karkowsky, MD, was the psychiatric consultant to the Plattsburgh, NY Air Force Strategic Air Command (SAC) Base when I was stationed there (1965–1967). By default I became the acting psychiatrist under his supervision. He opened my eyes, not so much to traditional psychiatric concepts, but to how to "read" people, to pick up clues of body language, and to understand that what is not discussed is as important, or more so, than what is discussed. Thanks to his example, I no longer sit behind a desk (a sign of importance and distance), but across from my patients. This communicates an equality and concern vital to the doctor-patient relationship.

Finally, to Sir Arthur Conan Doyle, a failed London eye doctor, who gave us Sherlock Holmes, a wonderful tutorial on accurate observation and deductive reasoning.

—Neil Raff

Preface

What does it mean to be normal?

What does it mean to be healthy?

The answers to these questions are not set in stone. They continue to evolve as our understanding of ourselves and health changes with new discoveries.

Many health values, or readings, that were considered normal only a few decades ago are now known to be erroneous. For example, physicians once regarded a blood pressure level of 140/90 as being on the high end of normal—still within the safety zone, in other words. Today, we know this is not true, and that the risks associated with high blood pressure begin with readings above 120/80.

Similar changes in values have occurred with regard to blood sugar levels. Not too long ago, a fasting blood sugar level of 140 was considered safe. Now, that level has been lowered to a fasting blood sugar of 100, and recent evidence suggests that even that level may still be too high.

Another significant example of how our understanding of what constitutes health has changed is presently occurring in the field of cardiology. Until recently, as a result of research dating back to the mid-20th century, cardiologists and other physicians regarded elevated blood cholesterol levels to be a primary risk factor for heart disease, including heart attack and stroke. More recently, however, many of us in the medical field have come to understand that it is not a patient's cholesterol reading, per se, that is the issue, but whether or not cholesterol in the patient's bloodstream has become oxidized (a process that is akin to rust). For this reason, in addition to monitoring their patients' cholesterol levels, more and more doctors now examine markers such as C-reactive protein (CRP) levels, to screen their patients for signs of chronic inflammation, a telltale sign of oxidation in the body.

Another major area in which our understanding of medicine and health has shifted in recent years has to do with genetics. It was once universally accepted that one's genes determined whether or not a person would develop various diseases, including cancer. While there is no doubt that genes certainly do play a role in determining a person's health, ongoing research by scientists is now showing us that, in many cases, the genes themselves may not be as important as we once believed. What may matter more is how those genes are influenced by internal (thoughts, emotions, and beliefs) and external (environmental toxins, diet) factor. This discovery indicates that how and why genes become activated (triggered) or deactivated (shut down) is more predictive of both health and disease than a patient's genetic profile alone. And it has led to the creation of an entirely new field of scientific inquiry known as *epigenetics*—the study of how genes are influenced for better or worse.

Just as science is changing our understanding of health and disease, so too is the new wave of scientific discoveries changing how physicians, including myself, understand and practice medicine. In my case, one example of this has to do with the pH levels of the human body, which is the subject of this book. In medical school, I was taught that blood pH stayed within a very narrow range, and did not shift beyond that except in extreme cases of disease. This is true, and as a result, I did not concern myself with my patient's pH levels when I first began practicing medicine except in cases of medical emergencies. After all, I reasoned, blood pH is fixed and, with the exception of such emergencies, it cannot and will not change.

Based on my understanding of pH at the time, it did not occur to me to consider how diet and other lifestyle factors might impact the body's overall pH balance. While I certainly understood and emphasized the importance of a proper diet for good health, and still do, back then I was unaware of how the foods and drinks we consume can influence bodily pH once they are digested and metabolized. Fortunately, however, as a growing body of studies about the impact of diet on pH began to come to my attention, my interest in pH levels in relationship to health and disease was piqued. As my interest grew, I was surprised, and then excited, by how powerful a diet that supports the body's mechanisms for regulating its pH levels can be as a tool we all can use to maintain and improve our health and reduce our risk of illness.

This new understanding on my part led me to reevaluate what I'd been taught in medical school—that, under most circumstances, blood pH is fixed and cannot be changed. I asked myself, Is this really so? The answer, I now know, is still yes, but that alone is not enough as it relates to how I now practice medicine. What must also be taken into account is what the body has to do to maintain its pH blood level. As this book explains, the answer to that question very much depends on both one's diet and one's lifestyle.

Of equal importance, in my view, is the rate of change when it comes to shifts in pH. To understand what I mean by this, consider what happens when we our exposed to bright sunlight. If our exposure is gradual and not overlong, we develop a healthy tan. But if our exposure is abrupt and long, we develop sunburn and increase our risk for skin cancer.

Similarly, should we move to an area situated at a higher altitude than we are used to, it will generally take our bodies three to four weeks before we are able to be fully acclimated to the thinner air. Yet, for the most part, we won't suffer any negative health consequences beyond, perhaps, an initial shortness of breath or labored breathing. But if we should hyperventilate (over breathe), within one to two minutes we will find ourselves getting lightheaded, dizzy, and feeling numb all over. That's because we will have too quickly increased our blood pH in that short period of time.

The above examples provide clues to how our bodies go about maintaining pH levels. The key point to remember is that it is far more difficult for our bodies to cope with a rapid and regular intake of foods and drinks that negatively impact pH levels (primarily foods and drinks that create a buildup of acids in the body that have to be neutralized), than it is when your meals consist primarily on non-acidifying foods and drinks.

Much scientific evidence points to increasing acidity in our nation's croplands and our environment in general (remember acid rain?), and thus in many of the foods we eat. This shift has had a harmful effect on the chemistry of our bodies, and on our health. This book provides a program of diet and life style to reverse this trend so that you can begin to move your body back to a more healthy pH and overall chemical balance.

—Neil Raff, MD

Introduction

Today, more than ever, it is obvious to most people that our nation is facing a health crisis that threatens to bankrupt us. Even with the advent of the Affordable Care Act, also known as "Obamacare," the cost of health care continues to rise, both in terms of treatment costs and insurance premiums. At the same time, more people in the US suffer from chronic, degenerative disease than ever before, while nearly half of our population is dangerously overweight or obese. While our politicians, economists, and health experts argue about how best to address these concerns, few, if any, seem to have any realistic long-term solutions.

Perhaps that's because they are overlooking the obvious. The truth is that the solution they are looking for does exists. It is a solution that isn't complicated, doesn't require billions of tax dollars, and doesn't need a giant bureaucratic overseer. What is that answer?

Good health. If fewer people needed pills to lower blood pressure, decrease cholesterol levels, or stimulate their love lives, think about the impact it would have on our health care system. If fewer people suffered from the severe pain of arthritis, rheumatism, and other degenerative diseases, think of how much emptier doctors' offices would be. And, if the number of people diagnosed with cancer and heart disease started to drop sharply, think of how much less sorrow and grief there would be in our lives.

The sad truth is that health is something the majority of people in this country are lacking. The incidence of chronic illness is at an all-time high. Just as alarming, even among people who don't suffer from any obvious disease symptoms, is that lack of energy seems to be epidemic, as well. Yet, paradoxically, at no time in history has such a wealth of health information been available to us, as evidenced by the abundant supply of books, newsletters, magazines, seminars, and web sites all devoted to providing health information. So why is it that, as a nation, we remain so unhealthy? And, more importantly, what can be done about it?

That's what this book is all about. We wrote it to answer these questions, and to empower you with the information you need to reclaim and maintain your health and vitality now and for the rest of your life. After years of careful research, study, and observation, we can say with absolute confidence that the solution to our health problems does exist, and it starts with the type of "medicine" that healers throughout history have recommended for more than 2,500 years—healthy food.

Your body is designed to be healthy. This is a scientific truth. And it *will* be healthy if you provide it with the right foods and the abundant supply of life-supporting nutrients they contain to repair and maintain itself. This fact has been known and taught by physicians and healers throughout the ages.

In recent decades, however, our understanding of what eating healthy means has changed thanks to the growing body of research focused on pH or acid-alkaline balance and the paramount role it plays in our health. Thanks to this research, we now know that eating healthy foods alone is not enough; we also need to eat them in the right proportions so that our bodies' pH levels are properly maintained. You will learn why this is so important in the pages ahead. Moreover, we will provide you with everything you need to know to create health-enhancing, pH-balancing meals quickly and easily.

But diet alone, no matter how healthy it may be, is rarely enough to completely provide you with adequate health. Think of your diet as the foundation upon which your health is built. Without such a strong foundation, long-term health simply is not possible. However, once that foundation is put in place, you still need to add the other elements that create the "house of health" in which you want to reside. These other elements are what make up your daily routine. Combined together, we call this living the *acid-alkaline lifestyle.*

No matter what state of health you may currently be in, if you apply the guidelines we will share with you, we guarantee that you will experience a noticeable difference in how well you feel. A bold claim, to be sure, but we make it with confidence, because we have witnessed how people from all walks of life have already experienced dramatic improvements in their health after implementing the very same principles you will discover in this book. Even if you are already healthy, these principles can help you.

In the pages that follow, you will not only learn how your body works, but also how you can begin to move it from a state of degeneration and fatigue into a state of regeneration and vitality. First, you will also learn about the foundational key—proper acid-alkaline balance, including its importance and how you can quickly begin to achieve and maintain it; why it is misunderstood or ignored by most health practitioners; and why unhealthy pH levels—a disruption of proper acid-alkaline balance—are at the root of all disease conditions.

Then we will guide you on how to most effectively create the acid-alkaline lifestyle for yourself and your loved ones. Throughout the rest of this book you will learn why this way of life is fundamental. Why the foods you eat are the key to good health. By knowing what foods to eat, how to prepare these foods, and when to eat them, you can take charge of your health once and for all. The following principles that will be addressed are fundamental to a healthy lifestyle.

- Why water may be the missing key to better health and more energy.

- The importance of nutritional supplements in today's ever-increasingly toxic world, and the nutritional supplement program we recommend for taking your health to the next level.

- How to improve your health simply by breathing properly, something most people don't pay attention to or know how to do.

- How to easily incorporate daily exercise into your lifestyle without having to spend a lot of time, money, or to use expensive exercise equipment.

- How to cope with stress with proven, easy-to-use self-care stress management techniques.

- The vital importance of adequate, restful sleep and how to ensure it.

Fortunately, the principles you are about to discover are easy to understand, and even easier to implement. By applying them to your daily life, you will be taking back control of your health and starting down the road to optimal vitality. No matter what health challenge you may presently be facing, you can improve it by adopting the guidelines that follow. This is our message to you: You don't have to be sick!

So, if you are ready to reclaim your health, turn the page and read on.

PART 1

Understanding Acid-Alkaline Balance

1

Acid-Alkaline Balance
What It Is and Why It Is So Vital to Your Health

A poor diet, lack of exercise, stress, environmental pollution—all of these and other factors are significant impediments to your overall well-being and must be addressed if good health is to be achieved and maintained. Yet, even when they are addressed, the health gains that are achieved will not be lasting if a much more basic factor remains overlooked, bringing your body back into balance—specifically, the acid-alkaline balance.

Unfortunately, it is this most vital aspect of health that is so often ignored by health care practitioners. Yet the concept of acid-alkaline balance is not a new discovery. In 1933, for instance, William Howard Hay, M.D., wrote a book entitled *A New Health Era*. In it, he wrote, "[W]e depart from health in just the proportion to which we have allowed our alkalis to be dissipated by introduction of acid-forming food in too great amount." Dr. Hay went on to write, "It may seem strange to say that all disease is the same thing, no matter what its myriad modes of expression, but it is verily so."

Arthur C. Guyton, M.D., regarded as a leading world authority on human physiology, echoed Dr. Hay's views a few decades later, when he wrote *The Textbook of Human Physiology*, a classic text that remains essential reading for today's class of medical students. In it, Dr. Guyton says, "[The regulation of hydrogen ion concentration is one of the most important aspects of homeostasis." In plain English, "hydrogen ion concentration" means pH, or the acid-alkaline balance, and "homeostasis" refers to the body's inherent self-regulating mechanisms, which seek always to maintain equilibrium, or balance, within all of the body's systems.

A balanced pH is one of the most vital factors necessary for achieving and maintaining good health. Too often, however, doctors ignore acid-alkaline balance except in cases of medical emergencies. For example, conventional medicine only recognizes alkalosis and acidosis when they reach an extreme life-threatening situation, such as diabetic coma or kidney failure (uremia), each of which are examples of extreme acidosis, or prolonged vomiting or muscle spasms, both of which are symptoms of acute alkalosis. Otherwise doctors typically pay little attention to pH. This is a mistake, one that can potentially lead to serious health problems for their patients.

In this chapter, you will learn why the acid-alkaline balance is so important to your health, and discover how an unbalanced pH can lead to disease. You will also learn how to determine the state of your own pH. Is your body in balance; are you too acidic; or are you too alkaline? Let's begin by learning more about what pH and acid-alkaline balance really mean.

WHAT IS pH?

Whether or not your body is in a state of acid-alkaline balance is determined by measuring pH. Your pH refers to the relative concentration of hydrogen ions in a solution, such as blood, urine, and saliva. The term itself was first defined in 1909 by a Danish biochemist named Soren Peter Lauritz Sorenson. Since that time it has been used to measure the acidic, alkaline, or neutral properties of various solutions and compounds. In terms of health, pH is a measurement of the acid-alkaline ratio of the body's fluids and tissues. When this ratio is balanced, good health results. When it is imbalanced—either too acidic or too alkaline—the body's internal environment is negatively impacted, setting the stage for disease to take hold.

pH, Acids, and Hydrogen ions in the Body

All acids in the body contain hydrogen atoms, the combination of which forms hydrogen molecules. *Molecule* is the term we use to denote the smallest quantity into which a substance can be reduced without losing any of its characteristics. When molecules containing hydrogen are dissolved in water and a hydrogen atom breaks off—a process known as *dissociation*—they create charged particles called hydrogen ions. Hydrogen ions are single, unstable protons that literally "hide" in the body's water molecules.

All acids in the body give off hydrogen ions when they are dissolved in water. In fact, this very property is what makes these substances acids. Any substance that reacts with acids is known as a *base,* and any base that dissolves in water is known as an *alkali.* Whether a substance is acidic or alkaline depends on the concentration of ions within it. The measurement of this concentration is called "potential for hydrogen," or pH for short. The pH scale of measurement ranges from 0 to 14, with 7 being neutral—neither acidic nor alkaline. Any measurement below 7 is considered acidic, while any measurement above 7 is considered alkcline. The greater the concentration of hydrogen ions in a substance, the more acidic it is.

The pH values are determined according to the concentration of hydrogen ions represented as moles per liter. (The term *mole* is short for *molecular weight.*) Pure water, which is considered neutral, has a concentration of hydrogen ions that equals 0.0000001 moles of moles per liter, or 10^{-7} moles per liter. By contrast, an extremely acidic substance might have a concentration of hydrogen ions as high as 0.01, or 10^{-2} moles per liter.

As you can see from these examples, concentrations of hydrogen ions are written as a power of 10. To indicate their pH values, we simply remove the base number 10 and the minus sign. Thus, a pH of 7 would be the value of pure (neutral) water, while a pH of 2 would indicate very high acidity. An increase of one point of pH is equal to a tenfold *decrease* in hydrogen ion concentration, while a decrease of one point of pH equals a ten-fold *increase* in hydrogen ion concentration.

The pH is measured on a scale of 0 to 14. A pH of 7 is considered neutral, while values below seven show a greater concentration of positively charged hydrogen ions compared to negatively charged ions. Conversely, a pH value greater than 7 indicates a higher concentration of negatively charged ions. A pH reading below 7 is an indication of acidity, and reading above 7 indicates an alkaline condition.

In order to thrive, your body's blood chemistry needs to be slightly alkaline. In a state of optimal health, the pH of your blood would be 7.365. When your pH blood reading moves too far below or above this number and remains that way, the inevitable result is that you will become sick. Some people who are chronically ill have a blood pH that is overly alkaline. However, the majority of people suffering from chronic illness suffer from an unbalanced blood pH that is far too acidic.

When this state of over-acidity becomes chronic, a number of serious threats to your health can arise. This occurs because the bloodstream fluids change to an environment that diminishes the body's internal oxygen supply and supports disease-producing microorganisms. Not all parts of the body operate within the same pH range, however. This is because, as Dr. Arthur Guyton pointed out in his *Textbook of Medical Physiology*, there are different levels of acidity and alkalinity in which your body's various organs, tissues, and fluids can function optimally. Examples of Dr. Guyton's findings are shown in Table 1.1 on page 11, which lists various body organs, tissues, and fluids and their respective pH range. In each of these areas of the body, numerous chemical and enzyme reactions occur. For these reactions to be performed as nature intended, a particular pH range is necessary. Small changes in pH levels can profoundly affect the body's overall function and energy levels.

As you can see from this table, both saliva and urine have a wide range of pH values, yet health can still exist as long as these ranges are not exceeded or diminished. Blood pH, on the other hand, must be maintained within a much narrower range for health to also be maintained, and this is why the blood pH read-

TABLE 1.1 HEALTHY pH VALUES OF THE HUMAN BODY	
BODY FLUIDS, TISSUES, AND ORGANS	HEALTHY PH VALUE
Brain	7.1
Blood	7.35 to 7.45
Heart	7.0 to 7.4
Liver	7.2
Saliva	6.0 to 7.4
Skeletal Muscle	6.9 to 7.2
Urine	4.5 to 8.0

ing is the most important determinant of your body's acid-alkaline balance.

HOW THE BODY REGULATES pH

Because appropriate pH levels are so vital to maintaining proper body function, nature designed a number of interrelated mechanisms that help regulate the acid-alkaline balance of your body's fluids, organs, and tissues. These mechanisms work in two ways: either by eliminating excess acid or by neutralizing acid by drawing upon the body's mineral stores. Let's examine how each of these self-regulating processes work.

Eliminating Acids

Elimination of acids is chiefly accomplished by the kidneys and lungs, and to a lesser extent, through the skin. Your kidneys play a vital role in helping to regulate blood pH, by helping to eliminate what are known as fixed or solid acids, such as uric and sulfuric acids. When pH levels become too acidic, the kidneys excrete additional hydrogen ions into the urine, while retaining extra sodium. This process filters fixed acids out of the bloodstream, diluting them so that they can be eliminated in the urine. Phosphate (a form of the mineral phosphorus) is required for this to occur, and if enough reserves are not available, the body draws phosphorus directly from its bones.

In cases of extreme acidity, the kidneys excrete increased hydrogen into the urine in an attempt to rid themselves of the acid. In cases where the body is too alkaline, this process is reversed, with the kidneys retaining more hydrogen and excreting extra sodium. When the buildup of fixed acids exceeds the kid-

Possible Indications of Changes in Urine Color and Odor

While changes in urine color and odor can often accompany excessive acid buildup in the body, such changes can also be due to other conditions, and may also be an indication of an underlying disease condition. Changes in urine odor can be due to dehydration (insufficient water intake), infection, or the over-consumption of nutritional supplements (particular B vitamins) or foods, such as asparagus, which is notorious for producing urine odor, especially among people who don't usually eat it. But strong urine odor can also be due to underlying illnesses, including diabetes, kidney stones, and urinary tract infections.

Changes in urine color can also be due to dehydration, particularly if the urine is cloudy or rust-colored. Urine color change can also occur as a result of over-exercise or exertion; eating certain foods, such as asparagus, beets, blackberries, borscht, or rhubarb; taking nutritional supplements, which can cause urine to become bright yellow or orange, or using medications, including laxatives. Changes in urine color can also be due to blood in the urine or various disease conditions, including bladder cancer, cirrhosis of the liver, diabetes, diarrhea, enlarged prostate (BPH), hepatitis (A, B, or C), jaundice, kidney cancer, kidney disease, kidney stones, pancreatic cancer, prostate cancer, prostatitis (prostate infection), urinary stones, or urinary tract infections. If changes in urine odor or color persist or are accompanied by other symptoms, seek prompt medical attention.

neys' maximum daily capacity for elimination, problems can occur. In cases of normal kidney function, signs that your body is too acidic include cloudy and/or rust-colored urine, and a noticeable urine odor. When acidic buildup is particularly high, a burning sensation can also accompany urination. It's important to note, however, that changes in urine color and odor can also be due to other factors, including various disease conditions. (See *Possible Indications of Changes in Urine Color and Odor* on page 12.)

As you breathe, your lungs also help to regulate acid-alkaline balance. During the breathing process, carbon dioxide combines with water in the blood to form a type of acid called carbonic acid. Respiration helps remove carbonic acid from the bloodstream, thus decreasing acidity. Your rate of respiration varies depending on how acidic or alkaline your body is. In conditions of over-acidity, your respiratory rate will tend to become faster, as your body attempts to remove higher levels of carbonic acid to help bring acid-alkaline levels back into balance. Similarly, in conditions of excess alkalinity, respiration rates tend to slow down, as the body seeks to retain acids to reduce alkaline levels. By learning how to regulate and deepen your breathing, you can help enhance your body's ability to deal with excess acidity via respiration. We will discuss this in more detail in Chapter 7.

The sweat glands in your skin also help to eliminate acids. As we perspire, acids are flushed out of your body. However, less acid is eliminated in this process compared to urination. On average, you eliminate nearly a quart of sweat every 24 hours, compared to about one and a half quarts of urine that is eliminated during the same period. In addition, smaller concentrations of acids are carried away by sweat than by urine. Body odor associated with perspiration is usually a strong indicator that your body is too acidic.

Neutralizing Acid Buildup

Neutralization of acids can occur during the digestive process and through cellular metabolism. When you eat a meal, as the foods you consume are digested, both the stomach and pancreas secrete substances that can affect acid-alkaline balance. The stomach secretes hydrochloric acid (HCl) to help the body breakdown food. This, in turn, causes the pancreas to secrete bicarbonate, a form of acid salt that neutralizes, or buffers HCL after it performs its function. If HCl is not neutralized, it can interfere with the pancreatic enzymes that are also necessary for proper digestion.

Usually, these secretions create temporary corresponding fluctuations in blood pH. But once the digestive process is complete, the blood pH soon returns to normal. However, poor diet, as well as the other factors can interfere with this process causing these secretions to become unbalanced.

The most common symptom of this imbalance is heartburn, due to over-acidity. Often we take heartburn medications, such as Tums, Rolaids, and Alka-Seltzer, for this problem, which only offer temporary relief of these symptoms and do not address its underlying causes. Studies indicate that when these antacids are used on a regular basis, they can actually make the problem worse. They can disrupt the acid-alkaline balance, and interfere with your body's ability to properly absorb folic acid, vitamin B12, and many of the minerals essential for good health.

Ironically, the ads you see on TV for heartburn medications imply that heartburn is due to excess production of stomach acid (HCl). In actuality, this isn't true. Research published as early as the 1960s, in peer-reviewed medical journals such as *Lancet*, indicated that in most cases of abnormal HCl production, *too little* HCl is being produced, not *too much*. This is especially true as we get older. When HCl is lacking, certain foods, especially proteins, are only partially digested, which can lead to fermentation of undigested food particles in the stomach, resulting in stress and inflammation of the small intestine, which, if it persists, can interfere with your body's ability to absorb and metabolize nutrients. But lack of HCl production is not the only potential cause of over-acidity.

Too little bicarbonate production by the pancreas can also cause over-acidity. Diarrhea, which diminishes the body's bicarbonate supply, and vomiting, which can result in loss of stomach acid, can also cause problems. However, the most common underlying culprit is poor diet—often accompanied by eating too much or eating too fast (gulping down meals without allowing the food to be properly chewed and digested). In the vast majority of cases, when dietary habits improve, heartburn and digestive-related issues resolve themselves automatically. You will learn more in Chapter 4 about what steps you can take to ensure that you are eating the foods best suited for maintaining a healthy acid-alkaline balance.

Not only is the body blessed by nature with various methods of controlling normal blood pH levels, it also has similar inherent mechanisms designed to regulate the acid-alkaline balance within each individual cell. This is primarily accomplished in two ways. In the first method, regulation is achieved by pumps within the cell membrane. It is through these pumps that hydrogen molecules enter and exit the cells. In order for this process to properly occur, phosphorus and magnesium are required. When they are not readily available, the body will pull them from bone and/or various organs. If forced to do so on a regular basis, our body will eventually move out of homeostasis, setting the stage for illness to occur. In the second method of cellular regulation, internal cellular pH levels are maintained by the cells themselves, which alter chemical reactions depending on how much or how little hydrogen needs to be produced.

In addition to these methods, when pH imbalances are prolonged, the body will seek to compensate for them by drawing out various minerals, including calcium, magnesium, potassium, and sodium, from bones and organs. It does so in order to neutralize the buildup of acids and then safely eliminate them. But if the body has to resort to such methods for long periods, it places itself under internal strain. Such stress of this nature can eventually create great damage to the body, causing premature aging, excessive weight gain, lack of energy, and impaired digestion and elimination, among a host of other conditions.

HARMFUL EFFECTS OF pH IMBALANCES

As we have seen, when pH levels become imbalanced for prolonged periods of time, your body's internal environment will
become either too acidic or too alkaline. In the vast majority of
cases, over-acidity or *acidosis,* is the problem. Many health practitioners who do address pH imbalance only focus on acidosis
because of how prevalent it is today. But for some people, over-
alkalinity, also known as *alkalosis,* is at the core of their health
problems.

Although conditions of alkalosis are far rarer than acidosis,
they too can cause various health problems. According to Dr. Guyton, alkalosis is primarily caused by over-consumption of drugs
that produce an alkalizing effect in the body, especially the anti-
heartburn preparations discussed previously, as well as prescribed
ulcer medications. Alkalosis can also occur as a result of chronic
diarrhea or vomiting, both of which can result in the loss of HCl
and other acids. When alkalosis sets in, your body is deprived of
the acids that are necessary to maintain proper balance.

The major side-effect of alkalosis is over-excitability of the
nervous system. According to Dr. Guyton, "This effect occurs both
in the central nervous system and in the peripheral nerves [all
nerves located outside of the central nervous system], but usually
the peripheral nerves are affected before the central nervous system. The nerves become so excitable that they automatically and
repetitively fire even when they are not stimulated by normal
stimuli." This, in turn, can lead to a condition known as *tetany.*
This disorder is characterized by muscle spasm and/or muscle
cramps that can be quite painful. Interestingly, tetany can also be
caused by hyperventilation or "over-breathing." As you learned
earlier in this chapter, breathing is one of the ways that your body
rids itself of excess acids. When we hyperventilate, too many acids
can be eliminated, leading both to tetany and a temporary state
of alkalosis.

If the peripheral nerves continue to be affected by alkalosis,
eventually the central nervous system can become affected as

well. Although the likelihood of this happening is not great, when it does occur the consequences can be serious. The most common symptom is extreme nervousness due to the over stimulation of the central nervous system itself. In extreme cases, convulsions can also occur. People who suffer from epilepsy can experience seizures if their bodies become too alkaline. Such people would do well to avoid alkaline drugs or only use them under the strict supervision of their physician.

THE RELATIONSHIP BETWEEN ACID-ALKALINE BALANCE AND THE HEALTH OF YOUR CELLS

Scientists estimate that our bodies are composed of approximately 100 trillion cells, which are divided into 150 different types. These include nerve cells, blood cells, bone cells, muscle cells, organ cells, and so forth—each performing specialized tasks. Collectively, all of these cell groups work in tandem with each other to govern, orchestrate, and carry-on all of your body's life-sustaining functions, including self-regulation, self-repair, and self-renewal. These groups of cells work well so long as they receive an adequate supply of oxygen, water, vitamins, minerals, enzymes, essential fatty acids, and other essential materials that serve as their building blocks. However, when this supply of nutrients is diminished or cut off, it sets the stage for disease and premature aging to occur.

It is, therefore, at the cellular level that all disease begins. Once disease takes hold in the cells, it then begins to attack various organs and body systems, such as the immune and endocrine systems. Proper acid-alkaline balance is vital for the healthy function of all aspects of the body's biochemistry. Your body's cells communicate with each other through a complex interaction of electrical, chemical, and hormonal processes. For proper communication between cells to take place, a slightly alkaline pH (7.365) in the blood is absolutely essential. Otherwise, cellular communication can become interrupted. When this happens, the stage is set for disease to occur.

As you learned above, the most common type of pH imbalance is over-acidity or acidosis. The acid waste products produced by your body each and every day cannot be adequately eliminated when the pH of your blood falls into a chronically acidic state. As your body struggles to restore proper pH balance excess wastes start to overwhelm the system. In the process, these waste products can severely compromise the integrity of your cells, and can seriously impair their ability to function properly due to toxic overload. In addition, the waste products prevent the cells from receiving enough oxygen and nutrients, and they can disrupt their ability to communicate with each other.

Earlier in this chapter we examined some of the ways in which your body attempts to restore pH balance by eliminating and neutralizing excess acid buildup. If these mechanisms are unable to completely neutralize accumulated acids, the next step your body takes is to divert the acids away from vital organs. When this occurs, your body will start storing the acids in your tissues, joints, and bones. If this process continues, you are likely to develop joint and skeletal problems, such as osteo- and rheumatoid arthritis, and possibly gout. In addition you can develop skin conditions, such as dermatitis and eczema, and/or tissues problems, such as chronic fatigue and fibromyalgia.

Though these conditions can certainly be debilitating, they are not life-threatening. But if acidosis continues, eventually toxic acids will start to be stored in vital organs. This can lead to far more serious health problems, including diabetes, heart disease, and cancer. To a large degree, the type of disease you develop depends upon which of your organs are most susceptible to being impaired by these toxic wastes. For example, if your gastrointestinal tract is most susceptible, you may be at increased risk for inflammatory conditions in your GI tract. But if the acids, instead, target the myelin sheath, which serves as a protective layer of insulation around the nerve fibers of the central nervous system, the nerve impulses from the brain to muscles can be impaired, resulting in conditions such as neuritis, peripheral neuropathy, and disturbances of the autonomic nervous system. *The name of the disease you develop is not as important as the underlying cause—toxic buildup of acid wastes due to a chronic state of acidosis in your bloodstream.*

What happens to the cell membranes may further compound this downward spiral to ill health. As acid wastes continue to accumulate, the cells' ability to absorb oxygen and nutrients eventually becomes blocked. This occurs as the cell membranes are coated over with the acidic waste products, losing their permeability. If this process is unchecked, eventually the cell membranes will start to harden and solidify. In response, the cells spill out additional waste products in the form of carbon dioxide and lactic acid. This increases the acidic environment, dropping pH levels even further.

If this process is not reversed, the cells become covered in extra-cellular waste and start to die off prematurely. Premature cell death is followed by the decay of the body's tissues and organs. As this occurs, bacteria, fungi, molds, parasites, and other pathogens, all of which thrive in states of acidosis, begin to feed on these diseased areas in the body. As they do, they produce additional waste products that further reduce pH levels, and create an even greater burden on the body.

To better understand this process, picture what happens when a penny is dropped into a vat of acid. Almost immediately, the acid starts to corrode the penny. Eventually, this corrosion will completely eat away at the penny, and the acid solution will become a stagnant, murky chemical swamp. In much the same way, acidosis, left unchecked, corrodes the body from the inside out. In the process, it disrupts and impedes all of the body's internal functions, including immune response, circulation, digestion, hormone production, and neurologic function. All of this leading to various states of disease.

MEDICINE'S FAILURE TO ADDRESS ACID-ALKALINE IMBALANCES

Doctors all too often ignore the steady decline in the body's organs and their various functions that results from imbalanced pH. This helps to explain why modern medicine continues to have such a poor success rate when it comes to reversing chronic disease as opposed to merely managing symptoms. And this problem is further compounded by the fact that the very drugs prescribed by physicians to manage chronic disease symptoms actually add to the body's acidic burden.

Most pharmaceutical drugs, especially antibiotics, are acid-producing by their very nature. Using them to treat health conditions that are primarily caused by over-acidity in the body is like trying to extinguish a fire by lighting matches. Although pharmaceutical drugs absolutely have their place—especially when they are used to treat acute, life-threatening disease conditions—their prolonged use for non-acute, chronic conditions will invariably only serve to make the patients' problems worse. So for all those people who take pharmaceutical drugs on a prolonged basis, it is no wonder that they develop complications far beyond their original health complaints. Drugs prescribed to manage the symptoms of these complaints, combined with the state of acidosis that already exists, will invariably lead to further deterioration in the body.

If we are to succeed in resolving our nation's growing health crisis, we must look towards a solution that provides us with real answers; answers that can restore and maximize health. If we can understand that most major chronic degenerative diseases we are faced with today are primarily the result of unrecognized stages of acidosis and nutritional deficiencies, we can begin to see and understand how our immune systems are compromised. Pharmaceutical drugs are certainly capable of relieving pain and suppressing symptoms. However, since they are neither alkalizing nor nutritive, they do not address the core problem—they only encourage it. And, it is unlikely that our medical system will radically shift its focus to understanding and treating the real *causes* of disease. Change will only arise when patients demand a change in the system. In the meantime, it is up to each of us to learn to take better responsibility for our health, and to do all that we can to enhance it. The guidelines you are learning about in this book can help you go a long way to achieving these goals.

THE ACID-ALKALINE DEBATE

Although an ever-growing number of physicians and other health specialists now recognize the importance of acid-alkaline balance to their patients' good health, many health professionals still continue to dismiss the role that an alkalizing diet plays in maintaining and improving health due to a variety of misconceptions.

Food's Impact on Blood pH Levels

Perhaps the most common such misconception is that foods, once they are eaten and metabolized, have little impact on blood pH levels. Thus, they conclude, diet, regardless of whether or not it is alkalizing, has little effect on people's overall pH status and how well they are. Another common rationale used to dismiss acid-alkaline-balancing diets is the body of research pointing to the health benefits of the so-called "Caveman" or Paleolithic Diet, which emphasizes the consumption of acidifying foods such as meat, poultry, fish, and eggs.

But, as noted pH expert Dr. Susan Brown points out, experts who question the impact of food on the body's pH often base their views solely on the fact that the human body, including its organs and bloodstream, is designed to control acidity. As we pointed out above, the ideal pH for blood is approximately 7.35. (Specifically, healthy blood in the arteries has a pH between 7.35 to 7.45 due to its oxygen content, while healthy blood in the veins has a pH between 7.31 to 7.41 because of its greater carbon dioxide content.) These ranges are slightly alkaline and your body is constantly making adjustments in order to maintain them.

The key point to remember here is that your body can incur a high cost if it has to regularly compensate for a daily diet that has an overall acidifying effect once it is metabolized. That's because such a diet results in an ongoing buildup of acids within your body that it must deal with using its inherent protective mechanisms that neutralize acid. When these mechanisms are called upon over a long period of time, eventually various systems in the body become compromised. Over time, this sets the stage for disease, since even small changes in pH balance can profoundly and negatively affect your body's overall function and energy levels.

One example of this involves your body's enzyme system. All chemical reactions in your body are initiated by enzymes, all of which function in a very narrow pH range. If that pH range were to change for any length of time, neither the enzymes nor the chemical reactions they initiate would be able to function properly. Although biological systems might not completely fail, suboptimal cellular metabolism functioning could still ensue. This is one of the reasons why it is vitally important to follow an alkalizing diet that does not create a chronic buildup of acids in the body. This problem can largely be avoided by following the dietary recommendations we make in this book, which is something the skeptics seem not to appreciate or understand.

Protein-Rich Foods

Another popular misconception about achieving acid-alkaline balance through diet is that protein-rich foods, especially animal-derived products such as meats, fish, and poultry, are somehow unhealthy and should be avoided. Some proponents of acid-alkaline balance go so far as to insist that it can only be achieved through a vegetarian or vegan diet. This is not true.

However, when eating animal-derived foods, it is always a good idea to consume only organic, grass-fed, free range animal products and wild-caught fish, just as it is to consume organic fruits and vegetables. (For more, *see* page 59).

Proteins are the building blocks of every tissue in your body and are required by our cells throughout their lifespan in order for our cells to be able to repair and maintain their individual functions. In fact, every cell in your body contains protein, and it is a major component of the skin, bones, muscles, organs, and glands. Protein is also found in nearly all body fluids, including blood. Protein is essential for growth, for cell repair, the production of new cells, and even the buffering of acids. Without an adequate supply of dietary protein, none of these functions can be performed properly. That's because protein foods contain essential amino acids, which can only be supplied through diet since the body cannot manufacture them on its own.

When it comes to protein foods, the first thing to keep in mind is that only the intake of excessive protein ends up being acid-forming. The protein we use in daily maintenance and repair are fully used and do not leave an acid residue. So while it is true that excess protein-rich foods can create an acid load in the body once they are metabolized, that does not mean that a healthy and balanced amount of protein should be avoided. In fact, the opposite is true. It is not necessary to follow a vegetarian or vegan diet. Many people, in fact, cannot thrive on such diets and require a certain amount of animal-derived protein foods in order to optimally function.

On the other hand, research does show that eating protein foods excessively, without adequate alkalizing foods to counterbalance them, can indeed contribute to health problems over time, including heart disease, cancer, osteoporosis, and kidney disease. The key, as with all things related to health, is moderation and balance. Most people can obtain all of their protein needs by consuming between 50 to 60 grams of protein each day. Even higher intakes can be beneficial if accompanied by sufficient alkali mineral food and supplement dietary components. Overall, moderate protein intake, along with following the overall dietary recommendations that you will find in Chapter 4, will provide you with all of the important health benefits protein foods provide, while neutralizing their acid load.

Paleolithic Diet

Finally, there is the question of the Paleolithic, or ancestral diet, for which there is indeed a growing body of evidence showing that such a diet can offer health benefits. Doesn't such a diet contradict the acid-alkaline theory? Once again, the answer is no. First off, only some of the diets our ancestors consumed were high in animal protein. For example, in one recent study of the net acid load of 159 hypothetical pre-agricultural diets, 87 percent were found to be base-producing, meaning non-acid-forming. This is in contrast to our diet today which had been found by the same researchers to be highly acid-forming. Additionally, two early proponents of the Paleolithic diet, Melvin Konner, MD, PhD and S. Boyd Eaton, MD, now suggest that the acid- alkaline impact of the Paleolithic diet was in some cases alkaline, compared to the contemporary Western diet, which is excessively acidic.

Further, despite the high amounts of protein-rich foods that some of our ancestors consumed, such high protein foods, by themselves, are not what provide the health benefits that are now attributed to the Paleolithic diet. For, in addition to protein foods, the Paleolithic diet was high in vitamins, minerals, antioxidants, fiber, phytonutrients, and low in sodium while devoid of refined sugar, refined grains, and synthetic foods of any kind. These diets also contained abundant amounts of alkalizing foods (primarily roots, plants, nuts, seeds, and fruits), which is well in line with our own recommendations. Also significant is the fact that the diet of our ancestors was for thousands of years very high in potassium and very low in sodium chloride (salt), while the standard Western diet today contains high amounts of sodium chloride and is very low in potassium. The human body's kidney system and pH balance systems, in order to function properly, are both very dependent on a diet that is high potassium and low in sodium. Even further, sodium chloride as used today has now been found to be acid-forming in its own right, all by itself.

All of the above factors appear to be overlooked by skeptics of acid-alkaline-balancing eating plans, which is why so much confusion and debate still exists around this issue. Even so, the science is clear. As Dr. Brown states, "In sum, a nutrient-dense diet—which contains all the protein you need, along with plenty of alkalizing foods—can, indeed, help your body maintain a beneficial acid-alkaline balance. This, in turn, will provide a life-supporting environment for optimum physiological functioning." (You will learn how to create such a diet for yourself in Chapter 4.)

CONCLUSION

You now have a better understanding about how and why maintaining a proper acid-alkaline balance is so crucial to your health. In addition, you now know the steps your body takes to regulate pH levels in your body, especially within your bloodstream, as well as the toll that is placed on your body when these mechanisms are regularly drawn upon. And you now know the important role diet plays in helping you achieve and maintain this balance.

Yet poor diet alone is not the only cause of acid-alkaline imbalance. In the next chapter, you will discover what these other causes are, as well as why the eating habits of so many Americans today is a primary cause of our nation's epidemic of chronic, degenerative disease. To find out more, keep reading.

2

Causes and Effects of Acid-Alkaline Imbalance

As you learned in Chapter 1, when your body's pH levels become imbalanced over periods of time your body's maintenance and repair mechanisms are negatively impacted. Unless addressed, this sets the stage for disease to take hold. In fact, nearly all health conditions can be said to be due, at least in part, to prolonged acid-alkaline imbalance. In this chapter, you will discover more of why this is so and how such imbalances pose a threat to your overall health. First, though, let's examine the primary causes of acid-alkaline imbalance.

THE PRIMARY CAUSES OF ACID-ALKALINE IMBALANCE

There are four main factors that can disrupt acid-alkaline balance. Without question, the primary one is poor diet, but other factors can also exacerbate this problem, especially chronic stress, poor respiration, and poor sleep. Let's explore each of them in turn.

The Relationship Between Food and pH Balance

All of the foods you eat, once they are digested and metabolized (literally burned down), leave a residue of ash in your body. Depending on the type of food you eat and its mineral content, the ash residue will either be acidic, alkaline, or neutral. Foods that produce an acidic ash residue have an acidifying effect on the body and lower pH levels. Foods that leave an alkaline effect have the opposite effect, being alkalizing and raising pH levels. Foods that produce a neutral ash residue have little to no effect on pH levels. Generally speaking, foods eaten raw tend to also produce an alkalizing effect on pH levels, compared to cooked foods, which typically are acidifying in nature.

It is important to note that the acidifying, alkalizing, or neutral effects produced by the foods you eat are far more significant, in terms of your health, than the foods' inherent pH values prior to their consumption. For example, a number of foods that are acidic in nature, such as certain citrus fruits and vinegars, actually produce an alkalizing effect on the body after they are digested and metabolized. Not all acidic foods are acidifying when eaten, nor are all alkaline foods alkalizing when consumed. Therefore, knowing the effect a food will have on your pH levels is the key to choosing your foods wisely.

Ironically, the acidifying and alkalizing effects of foods are too often ignored by dieticians and nutritionists who focus solely on foods' nutrient content. Nutrients are, of course, essential to good health. But when pH levels are imbalanced, proper absorption and utilization of nutrients is interrupted, eventually resulting in nutritional deficiencies.

The same principles apply to the beverages you drink each day. Pure, filtered water has a pH value of approximately 7.0, making it an ideal beverage since its consumption results in a neural net pH load inside the body. By contrast, tap water typically has an acidifying effect inside the body, while various mineral waters are alkalizing. (You will learn more about water and its important health benefits in Chapter 6.) Other beverages can be either acidifying or alkalizing, as well.

The typical American diet consists primarily of foods that create an acid load once they are consumed and metabolized. Many beverages common to such a diet, such as soda, alcohol, coffee, and commercial juices and teas, add to this acid load. As we discussed in Chapter 1, to compensate for and neutralize this acid buildup, your body employs a variety of mechanisms in order to keep its pH levels, especially that of the blood, within their proper range. Having to take such measures on a consistent basis diverts energy away from your body's many other health-maintaining functions. Eventually, the burden created by ongoing consumption of overly acidifying foods and drinks takes a toll on your body's various repair mechanisms, leading to impaired health.

This basic fact continues to be ignored by most physicians, largely because their medical training is severely lacking when it comes to educating them about diet and nutrition. As a result, their patients are never told how simply shifting from their current eating habits to a diet that is more supportive of acid-alkaline balance can begin to quickly make important and lasting positive changes in their overall health.

How Stress Impacts Acid-Alkaline Balance

Although we all experience times of acute or fleeting stress as a normal part of our daily lives, with little to no impact on our health, chronic, unresolved stress is a much different matter. As it perpetuates, it can negatively impact health in a variety of ways. Physicians have long recognized, for instance, that chronic stress reduces immune function and increases susceptibility to harmful infectious disease conditions. Chronic stress has also been linked to an increased risk for both heart disease and cancer. It has also been shown to negatively affect your body's endocrine system, which is responsible for the production and regulations of hormones, leading to adrenal fatigue, as well as imbalances in the thyroid and pituitary glands. The relationship between chronic stress and various disease conditions also often results in a vicious cycle in which stress leads to illness and the illness creates additional levels of stress.

All of these facts are well-known by physicians and other health care providers. *What is less well-known is that chronic stress disrupts acid-alkaline balance and can make your body more acidic.* The explanation behind this fact has to do with one of the most important, yet often overlooked minerals in your body—magnesium.

Along with calcium and phosphorous, magnesium is one of the minerals that the body draws upon in order to buffer acid buildup, and is also the most abundant mineral in the brain. Unlike these other minerals, magnesium stores in the body are quickly depleted by chronic stress. Chronic stress results in a steady drain of magnesium, in much the same way that a leak in your car's gas line will eventually drain it of gasoline.

This analogy is more apt than it may seem at first. Just as gasoline is the fuel your car needs to operate, so too is magnesium the primary nutrient that your body uses to create and utilize energy. That's because magnesium is essential for the production of ATP (*adenosine triphosphate*) within the mitochondira, the energy factories inside each of the trillions of cells that make up your body. Lack of magnesium not only results in a lack of bodily energy and negatively impacts one of the primary mechanisms your body uses to neutralize acidity in your body, but it also leads to an increased production and release of your body's stress hormones. This further exacerbates the vicious cycle between stress and disease. Think of it this way: Stress increases the likelihood of disease *and* depletes your body's magnesium stores. Without enough magnesium, your body loses one of its main acid-neutralizing minerals *and your body's* cells cannot produce all of the energy it needs to combat disease. This allows both acidity and disease to gain greater footholds inside your body, which, in turn leads to even more stress! (In Chapter 5 you will learn more about the important health properties of magnesium, and in Chapter 8 you will learn how to better control and manage stress.)

Poor Respiration Causes More Acidity

You can live for weeks without food and days without water, but typically if you were stop breathing for more than a few minutes, you would die. Breathing is the single most important physical function we perform, yet almost all of us breathe inefficiently. Most of the time, we aren't even conscious of our breath, all the while breathing shallowly and depriving ourselves of the revitalizing energy that proper breathing can provide.

The primary purpose of breathing is to deliver oxygen to every cell of every tissue and organ in our bodies, while removing carbon dioxide. Oxygen's main role in the body is to produce the energy required for all of its function. This energy production occurs as a direct result of oxygen's interaction with ATP. When we breathe shallowly, our oxygen intake is reduced and ATP production is diminished as well.

But there is a second and equally important role that breathing plays. As we discussed in Chapter 1, respiration is one of the mechanisms your body uses to eliminate acid wastes in the body, thereby helping to maintain proper acid-alkaline balance. Habitual shallow breathing (hypoventilation) compromises this process and results in the accumulation of carbon dioxide in the body, which is then converted into carbonic acid, which causes acidosis. Thus, in addition to reducing the amount of energy your body needs to perform its tasks, improper breathing also results in an inefficient elimination of acid wastes, forcing your body to expend even more energy in other pH-balancing functions. The end result is both a drain on your body's available energy supply, and a buildup of acidity.

By simply learning how to improve the way you breathe, you can considerably improve your overall health, ensure that your cells thrive in an oxygen-rich, energizing state, and enhance your body's ability to more effectively maintain acid-alkaline balance. In Chapter 7 we share a variety of breathing exercises and techniques that will empower you to do so.

The Role That Sleep Plays in Maintaining Acid-Alkaline Balance

The importance of restful sleep cannot be overemphasized. Yet, as a nation, research continues to show that growing numbers of Americans fail to get all the sleep they need each night. Research also shows that lack of sleep and poor sleeping habits are directly related to a wide range of health problems, ranging from fatigue to type 2 diabetes, cancer, heart disease, and, possibly, Alzheimer's disease and dementia.

This is hardly surprising given the role that sleep is intended to play in keeping the body healthy. For it is while you are asleep that your body's repair mechanisms are most fully employed. In fact, recent research has even discovered that it is during sleep that the body is best able to eliminate toxins from the brain.

In addition to the many health benefits that regular, restorative sleep provides, a good night's sleep can be an important factor in your productivity, creativity, and enjoyment levels during the day and enhance your mood and cognitive function. Conversely, lack of sleep negatively impacts all of these areas of your life and also results in higher levels of stress. First, because poor sleep does not allow your body's repair mechanisms to fully do their job. Second, because lack of sleep also increases feelings of irritability, anxiety, and depression.

As we discussed above, when you are stressed, your body quickly depletes its stores of magnesium, one of the essential minerals that is called upon to buffer the buildup of acidity in the body. So, indirectly, poor sleeping habits impair your body's ability to keep acid buildup in check. Whereas a good night's sleep can enhance healing at all levels, lack of sleep exacerbates whatever health problems may be present, and increases the risk that you will develop other health problems in the future. All while it also interferes with your body's ability to maintain proper pH levels. Fortunately, there are a variety of sleep-enhancing steps you can easily take to improve the quality of your sleep. You will learn about them in Chapter 10.

Now that you have a better understanding of the primary causes of acid-alkaline imbalance, let's take a deeper look at the effects such imbalances can have on your health.

THE HEALTH-RAVAGING EFFECTS OF ACID-ALKALINE IMBALANCE

As we have seen, when pH levels become imbalanced for prolonged periods of time, your body's internal environment will become either too acidic or too alkaline. In the vast majority of cases, over-acidity or *acidosis,* is the problem. Many health practitioners who do address pH imbalance only focus on acidosis because of how prevalent it is today. But for some people, over-alkalinity, also known as *alkalosis,* is at the heart of their health problems.

Although conditions of alkalosis are far rarer than acidosis, they too can cause various health problems. According to Dr. Guyton, alkalosis is primarily caused by over-consumption of drugs that produce an alkalizing effect in the body, especially anti-heartburn preparations, as well as prescribed ulcer medications. Alkalosis can also occur as a result of chronic diarrhea or vomiting, both of which can result in the loss of hydrochloric acid (HCl) in the stomach and other acids. When alkalosis sets in, your body is deprived of the acids that are necessary to maintain proper balance.

The major side-effect of alkalosis is over-excitability of the nervous system. According to Dr. Guyton, "This effect occurs both in the central nervous system and in the peripheral nerves [all nerves located outside of the central nervous system], but usually the peripheral nerves are affected before the central nervous system. The nerves become so excitable that they automatically and repetitively fire even when they are not stimulated by normal stimuli." This, in turn, can lead to a condition known as *tetany.* Tetany is characterized by muscle spasms and/or muscle cramps that can be quite painful. Interestingly, tetany can also be caused by hyperventilation or "over-breathing." As you learned earlier, breathing is one of the ways that your body rids itself of excess acids. When we hyperventilate, too many acids can be eliminated, leading both to tetany and a temporary state of alkalosis.

If the peripheral nerves continue to be affected by alkalosis, eventually the central nervous system can become affected as well. Although the likelihood of this happening is not great, when it does occur the consequences can be serious. The most common symptom is extreme nervousness due to the over stimulation of the central nervous system itself. In extreme cases, convulsions can also occur. People who suffer from epilepsy can experience seizures if their bodies become too alkaline. Such people would do well to avoid alkaline drugs or only use them under the strict supervision of their physician. The dietary suggestions in Chapter 4 can also be beneficial.

Acidosis—The Primary Culprit

As we've mentioned, the majority of pH imbalances are related to acidosis, caused by an excess of acids in the body's internal environment. When acid buildup occurs to the point where the body is no longer able to successfully eliminate or neutralize these acids, a host of problems can occur, including illness and, potentially, even death. Other problems related to acidosis include accelerated aging, demineralization (loss of the body's mineral stores), fatigue, impaired enzyme activity, inflammation, organ damage, and the proliferation of harmful microorganisms such as bacteria, fungi, molds, yeasts (including Candida), and viruses.

Accelerated Aging

Accelerated or premature aging is all too common in our society. This condition can be due to a variety of factors, such as the accumulation of environmental toxins in the body, stress, and nutritional deficiencies. These factors can also affect pH levels, making your body more susceptible to disease. When your body's cells are continually exposed to an overly acidic environment, their cell structure can become altered, meaning that the cell's membranes lose their integrity. When viewed under a microscope, such cells, instead of being round and having noticeably strong walls, look bent and misshapen, with cell membranes that are thin and weak. In addition, their ability to function properly can be diminished, as can their ability to effectively communicate with other cells. Over time, this state of deterioration causes the cells to make "mistakes" as they seek to repair and regenerate themselves by manufacturing the proteins that are essential to this process.

Heat shock protein, in particular, can play a vital role in this process. Heat shock protein is a substance required by your body to facilitate cellular repair. It does so by aiding in the disposal of old or damaged proteins, while helping to build and transport new proteins. Acidosis impairs your body's ability to produce this substance. When less heat shock protein is produced as a result of over-acidity, this repair process can be seriously hampered. Such mistakes can trigger premature cell death as a result of the wrong proteins being manufactured, or because the right proteins are not being manufactured in their proper quantity. When this happens, shortages of substances such as collagen and elastin, both of which are essential for healthy, wrinkle-free skin, can arise, as well as impairment of your body's internal organ systems. All of which sets the stage for accelerated aging to occur, as well.

Acidosis can also impair proper brain function, which is also associated with aging. An overly acidic internal environment inhibits neuron function. Neurons are nerve cells that help initiate and conduct impulses from the brain. When neurons are unable to function properly, symptoms such as "brain fog," forgetfulness, and impaired mental acuity are more apt to occur. These are examples of a prolonged process of acidosis. By contrast, acute acidosis, as in diabetic acidosis, can cause coma, and even death, within a few hours time.

Demineralization

Your body draws upon its alkaline mineral stores in order to buffer or neutralize excess acids. While occasional withdrawal of these minerals is not likely to pose a problem, during chronic acidosis, the loss of such minerals, which include calcium, potassium, and magnesium, can pose serious health risks. Since these minerals are stored in all body tissues, their loss can potentially affect any of your body's organs. But it is your bones and teeth that are most especially affected by demineralization.

Dr. Susan Brown, a world-renowned expert in osteoporosis, points out that this condition is virtually nonexistent in cultures around the world that traditionally eat whole foods that help foster a balanced pH. In her book, *Better Bones, Better Body*, she states, "In our society, we consume a very imbalanced diet high in acid-forming foods. This imbalanced diet pushes us towards an acid state. Excessive and prolonged acidity can drain bone of calcium reserves and lead to bone thinning." As this thinning process occurs, our bones lose their flexibility increasing our risk for developing osteoporosis. We become far more susceptible to age-related fractures such as in the hip fractures. Rheumatism caused by inflamed joints can also develop, as can degeneration of spinal disks, potentially leading to conditions such as chronic back pain and sciatica.

Demineralization can also lead to tooth problems, since loss of calcium makes teeth more brittle and more susceptible to chipping. Your teeth may also start to experience sensitivity to hot and cold foods, and they may be more prone to develop cavities. Tooth decay and cavities, so prevalent in children today, are almost always caused primarily by a steady diet of acid-forming foods, such as the sugared cereals, sodas, and fast-food meals. Other common results of demineralization include dry and cracking skin, brittle and thinning hair, fingernails that crack or split easily, and bleeding and oversensitive gums.

Fatigue

Fatigue is one of the most common symptoms among people whose bodies start to become overly acidic. As over-acidity grows worse, so, too, does fatigue. The reason for this is simple and straightforward: Acidosis creates an internal environment in the body that is not conducive to optimal energy production. In an overly acidic environment, your body's blood supply of oxygen diminishes making oxygen less available to the cells, tissues, and organs.

Lack of oxygen interferes with your body's ability to carry out function like cell repair. It also impairs the ability of the mitochondria (your cell's internal "energy factories") to function. When the mitochondria are not well protected and properly fed— both consequences of acidosis and diminished oxygen supply— their ability to communicate with each other breaks down. This, in turn, compromises the mitochondria's energy production, leading to fatigue.

In an *anaerobic,* or low oxygen, environment (with the exception of the small intestine, which requires a relatively low oxygen environment to function properly), toxins and harmful microorganisms are also better able to flourish and proliferate. As they do so, they interfere with our body's ability to absorb and utilize nutrients, such as vitamins, minerals, and amino acids. This malabsorption of nutrients makes it much more difficult for your body to manufacture the enzymes, hormones, and numerous other biochemicals it requires for energy production, proper organ activity, and cellular repair. Blood sugar levels can also be affected, further affecting fatigue and impairing physical endurance. Microorganisms such as yeasts and fungus can also disturb electrolyte balance.

Electrolytes act as conductors of electricity throughout your body and play a vital role in cellular activity. When they become imbalanced, the normal flow of energy in your body is reduced. Acidosis impairs normal membrane function, interfering with the cells access to nutrients, which in turn diminishes all cells' ability to generate energy. If all of these factors are left unchecked, the result is chronic fatigue. By understanding this, and treating and resolving acidosis, you can also free yourself from fatigue and regain your energy.

Impaired Enzyme Activity

According to Edward Howell, M.D., author of *Enzyme Nutrition,* and the person responsible for pioneering the use of enzyme therapy in the United States, "Enzymes are substances that make life possible. No mineral, vitamin, or hormone can do any work without enzymes. They are the manual workers that build the body from proteins, carbohydrates, and fats. The body may have the raw building materials, but without the workers it cannot begin."

Thousands of different types of enzymes are manufactured by the body. Each one of them acts as a specific biological catalyst that is necessary for stimulating a particular biochemical reaction. Enzymes are necessary for every single process that the body performs including breathing, digestion, immune function, reproduction, proper organ function as well as speech, thought, and movement. But enzymes can only perform their multitude of tasks correctly within specific pH levels.

If these pH levels become imbalanced, as they do with acidosis, enzyme function becomes disrupted. In some instances, enzyme activity can cease altogether as a result of unhealthy pH levels. When this happens, illness occurs. Initially, the illness will usually be mild in nature, but it can quickly become more severe if nothing is done to restore the body's proper acid-alkaline balance. If this process is left unchecked, an illness can become life-threatening. If enzyme function is completely shut down due to unhealthy pH levels, eventually death will ensue.

Supplementing with digestive enzymes can help to safeguard against such health-sapping effects. For some people, this can be absolutely vital for restoring their health. Overall, however, enzyme supplementation will not achieve lasting positive results so long as your body remains in a state of chronic acidosis. Since it is the over-acidity that is the underlying cause of enzyme malfunction, it makes far better sense to restore the internal environment to its proper acid-alkaline balance in order to keep this problem from recurring.

Inflammation and Organ Damage

The excess acids that build up in the body due to an overly acidic pH are corrosive and can be damaging to the tissues and organs with which they come into contact. If not neutralized or eliminated, they can cause lesions and scarring of organ tissues, as well as, potentially, inflammation. The kidneys and skin can be particularly affected when the amount of acid is greater than they are designed by nature to get rid of. When the skin is affected, conditions such as hives, eczema, blotching, and itching can occur as a direct result of acidic sweat passing through the sweat glands. When excess acid buildup occurs in the kidneys, urination can become painful and the urinary tract can become inflamed, causing a painful, burning sensation during urination. Infection can also occur, leading to conditions such as cystitis, a type of bladder inflammation that is often accompanied by urinary tract infection.

Inflammation caused by acid buildup can occur anywhere in the body, leading to illnesses ending with "*-itis,*" a suffix used to indicate an inflammatory condition. Inflammation of the joints can cause arth*ritis,* for example, while inflammation of the nerves can lead to neur*itis,* inflammation in the lungs can cause bronchi*tis.* Inflammation of the gastrointestinal tract can result in col*itis* or enter*itis.* Another sign of inflammation in the body is burning pains in various other organs.

Tissues affected by acid buildup can not only be damaged, they can also become more susceptible to infection, due to lesions that allow invading microorganisms to more easily penetrate cells and tissues. Once such penetration occurs, these same microorganisms also have an easier time growing in numbers within the affected area.

Compounding this problem is the fact that acid buildup also impairs immune function. In a state of acidosis, production of white blood cells is diminished, and the white blood cells that are manufactured are of reduced strength. Since white blood cells play a vital role in your body's ability to target and destroy invading microbes, their diminished numbers and capacity resulting from excess acids in the body makes it easier for disease to take hold.

Proliferation of Harmful Microorganisms

When the pH of the blood remains consistently below 7.365, the bloodstream becomes a breeding ground for harmful microorganisms, much like a stagnant swamp. This happens because acidosis reduces the available oxygen supply in the bloodstream, and microorganisms thrive in the absence of optimum oxygen levels. In 1931, German researcher Dr. Otto Warburg was awarded the Nobel Prize for his discovery that cancer cells cannot exist in an oxygen-rich environment.

When the oxygen supply in the bloodstream is diminished, various cells within the body revert to what Warburg termed a "primitive" state, no longer deriving energy from oxygen, but from the fermentation of sugar in the form of glucose. This creates large amounts of lactic acid, a waste product of this fermentation. And it is this lactic acid that further diminishes available oxygen levels which disrupts the acid-alkaline balance. What's important to realize here is that it was the lack of oxygen that set this process in motion in the first place, and the lack of oxygen was caused by unhealthy acid levels in the bloodstream. By maintaining a balanced pH, all of this can be avoided.

The same anaerobic condition that causes cells to devolve and potentially turn cancerous, is also ideal for the proliferation of bacteria, fungi, molds, yeasts (including *Candida*), and viruses. These microorganisms also subsist by fermenting glucose, which under healthy conditions is used by your body to supply energy. In addition, they divert fats and proteins normally used by your body for regeneration and other functions, using them for their own reproduction. In this way, the microorganisms are able to spread throughout the body, targeting weak areas and breaking down tissue and interfering with the bodily processes that are essential for good health.

The most serious health problem posed by microorganisms is not the microorganisms themselves, but the waste products they produce during their life cycle. These excretions are also acidic. As they are dumped into your bloodstream, they further pollute your internal environment and invade your cells, to directly or indirectly produce a wide range of disease symptoms, all of which worsen as the microorganisms continue to proliferate.

Physical Symptoms of Microorganism Overgrowth

The most serious health problem posed by microorganisms is not the microorganisms themselves, but the waste products they produce during their life cycle. These excretions are also acidic. As they are dumped into your bloodstream, they further pollute your internal environment and invade your cells, to directly or indirectly produce a wide range of disease symptoms, all of which worsen as the microorganisms continue to proliferate. Among the more common of these symptoms are:

- bladder and urinary tract infections

- bleeding and/or receding gums

- candidiasis (*candida* yeast overgrowth)

- colds and flu

- cysts

- dizziness

- dry mouth

- finger and/or toenail fungus

- gastrointestinal disorders (acid reflux, bloating, colitis, constipation, diarrhea, enteritis, flatulence, halitosis, heartburn, hemorrhoids, indigestion, intestinal pains, ulcers)

- headache

- hyperactivity

- impaired immunity and greater susceptibility to infectious disease

- joint pain and/or muscle ache

- mental/emotional disorders (including antisocial behavior, anxiety, depression, irritability, mood swings, poor memory, and suicidal tendencies)

- skin problems (including dry skin, hives, itching, and skin rash)

Other Ways That Chronic Acidosis Harms the Body

In Chapter 1, we mentioned that critics of the importance acid-alkaline balance has to your overall health dismiss the need for following a diet and lifestyle that promotes such balance because of the body's own innate mechanisms designed to compensate for acid buildup. While these mechanisms most certainly exist and are indeed essential for keeping your body's pH levels (most especially your blood pH) balanced, if they are called upon to do so in an ongoing basis, before long your body's alkali mineral reserves will begin to be depleted. Such mineral depletion has many serious health implications.

Various scientific studies clearly demonstrate the toll that occurs within the human body when it is forced to consistently deal with chronic acidosis. The problems caused by doing, over time, can result in the following health problems:

- calcium loss, leading to reduced bone formation, bone thinning, and osteoporosis

- elevated levels of parathyroid hormone in the blood, which further impacts bone health, causing bones to become brittle and more susceptible to fractures

- loss of magnesium and potassium stores which, in turn, can lead to high blood pressure, chronic inflammation, chronic pain, and, in the case of magnesium loss, increased risk of heart disease

- unhealthy breakdown of protein (protein catabolism), resulting in loss of muscle mass and an increased risk of muscle wasting

- impaired protein metabolism, which negatively impacts your body's ability to repair its cells, tissues, and organs

- irritation of the bladder and urinary tract, resulting in an increased risk for bladder and urinary tract infections and painful or frequent urination

- disruption of your body's ability to produce growth hormone, insulin-like growth factor, and other pituitary hormones, causing hormonal dysfunction

- increased free radical production and oxidation, resulting in chronic inflammation, chronic pain, and suppressed immune function, as well as an increased risk of degenerative disease and premature aging

- increased risk of kidney stones and other kidney disorders

- increased fluid retention and fluid accumulation within body tissues

- disrupted intestinal bacteria, leading to digestive problems and an increased risk of yeast and fungal overgrowth within the gastrointestinal tract

- increased acidity of the mouth, causing an increase in oral bacteria and greater susceptibility to dental decay and gum disease

- increased toxicity in the liver and diminished liver function due to the buildup of acidic toxic wastes in the body

- over-production of stress hormones

- impaired thyroid function (hypothyroidism)

CONCLUSION

Having read this chapter, you now have a greater understanding as to the causes of acid-alkaline imbalances and, more importantly, you now know the extent that such imbalances can negatively affect your overall health, including the many serious disease conditions they can result in. Fortunately, there is much that you can do on your own to restore your body's acid-alkaline balance and, in the process, improve and maintain your health. The first step towards doing so lies in determining your current health status and your body's pH levels. You will learn how to do so in Chapter 3.

3

Are You Out of Balance?
Determining Your Body's pH Levels

The human body is a truly miraculous creation. It is designed to continuously maintain its healthy functioning through the process of homeostasis, its system of inherent self-regulating mechanisms, which seeks always to maintain the body's balance. Unfortunately, in today's modern world of stress, environmental pollution, and adulterated foods, it is becoming ever more challenging for our bodies to operate the way God and Nature intended. Due to all the stresses exerted on our bodies during the course of our day-to-day lives, homeostasis is becoming increasingly difficult to maintain. Once our bodies fall out of balance, a state of *disease* sets in, which, if left uncorrected, ultimately will lead to illness of one sort or another.

Many of us, however, tend to overlook the initial warning signs of this process, defining health as little more than the absence of actual disease. As a result, by the time disease symptoms are paid attention to it is often only after the disease itself has had an opportunity to stealthily progress to a state where medical intervention is necessary. It is precisely because so many people fail to pay attention to their bodies' early warning signs of imbalance that our health care system expenditures are primarily on medical treatments that could otherwise have been avoided.

One of the easiest, yet effective ways of monitoring your health status to prevent the onset of disease is by regularly checking your body's pH levels. First, though, let's take a moment to assess your current health status

HEALTH ASSESSMENT

Are you healthy? If you are reading this book without any obvious health complaints, most likely your answer to this question is yes. But is that really true? Physicians meet people all the time who tell them they are healthy and free of disease symptoms. Yet, when doctors examine them, many times it turns out that this isn't the case at all. While the patients may be correct in stating that they are not suffering from any obvious signs of illness, in point of fact, most of them admit to having some type of nagging complaint, such as lack of energy, minor, yet nagging, aches and pains, muscle tension or lack of flexibility, feelings of chronic stress, or an inability to get a good night's sleep.

If these nagging symptoms sound all too familiar to you, you should know that such complaints are common among millions of people in our nation today. All told, we have forgotten what being truly healthy actually means. Health is not merely a condition of being free of disease symptoms. It is a state of abundant energy and mental/emotional well-being. How close to this ideal are you?

What follows is a simple quiz that will enable you to discover how healthy you really are. As you go through it, note how many attributes of health you are experiencing now. At the same time, note how few of them you are enjoying. The more of them that reflect our current condition, the healthier you are. This test is by no means conclusive, but it will provide you with an easy way to assess your overall health in general terms. It can also help you determine what areas of your health you may need to work on.

The "How Healthy Are You" Quiz

For each point below, circle the number that most accurately is true for you at this present time. The number 1 refers to the least experienced, 3 as average, and 5 as the most. Make sure to answer honestly.

LEAST	OCCASIONALLY	MOST
1	2 3	4 5

1. You go through each day with abundant energy. ____

2. You have fall asleep easily and sleep deeply. ____

3. You awaken each morning feeling well-rested and ready to tackle the day. ____

4. You are within 20 pounds of your healthy body weight. ____

5. You feel fit and limber. ____

6. You are physically strong. ____

7. You feel physically attractive. ____

8. You have a positive overall mental outlook and can cope with your daily challenges. ____

9. You regularly experience joy and feelings of satisfaction. ____

10. You live and work in healthy environments that support your well-being. ____

11. You have strong and emotionally fulfilling bonds with your family and/or friends. ____

12. You feel connected to the world around you. ____

TOTAL POINTS ____

Now add up the number of points you have circled. If your total points fall below 30, your level of health may be easily comprised. If it falls between 30 to 50 points, you are healthier than most people, yet your level of health is subject to fluctuation. If, however, you have scored above 50 points, you have managed to create a stable health environment for yourself. If so, congratulations!

TESTING FOR ACID-ALKALINE BALANCE

Now that you have a better idea of your current health status, as well as a better understanding of the importance of pH to your health, determining your body's pH levels is an important next step you can take to learn whether or not you are in a state of acid-alkaline balance.

There are a number of tests available for measuring pH levels in the body. The first is the venous plasma pH test which can provide you with an accurate reading of your blood's pH level. The second is a self-test that can be easily done at home. It involves the use of pH strips. Although it does not provide specific pH measurements, it offers a strong indication of where you are in terms of acidic-alkaline balance.

Venous Plasma pH Test

The venous plasma pH test accurately measures the pH of your blood. It requires that you see a physician. Your doctor will withdraw a vial of blood from a vein in your arm, and then send the blood to a licensed laboratory for testing. Should you decide to have this test performed, be sure that you request that the measurement be made to the nearest one-hundredth of a percentage point, for example, 7.36 or 7.25, not 7.3 or 7.2. This will provide a more precise reading of your blood pH than if the measurement is only to a tenth of a percentage point.

Because of how important blood pH levels are to your overall health, you may want to consider making the venous plasma pH test part of your annual physical check-up. Since it is not commonly administered as part of such check-ups, be sure to ask your physician for it when you schedule your appointment. The additional cost is nominal (less than $100 depending on the lab your physician uses), and the information the test provides can literally be life-saving.

The pH Strip

You can also perform a simple home pH test using pH strips,

which are usually available at your local drugstore. Some health food stores may also carry them. These pH strips are made of litmus paper, which change color when it comes in contact with alkaline and acidic substances. Included with your purchase will be a color chart with corresponding pH values that will help you to gauge your pH.

You can use pH strips to test the pH levels of both your urine and saliva. However, since the pH of saliva can have a wide variance, we recommend testing your urine instead. As mentioned above, your kidneys are one of the organs used by the body to eliminate acids. When your body is in or near a state of acid-alkaline balance, urine pH will normally be 7.0 to 7.5 (pH strips do not measure pH values as closely as a blood pH test does). This indicates that your kidneys are excreting normal levels of acids. But when higher than normal amounts of acids are being eliminated, it means that your body is overly acidic. This will be reflected in the measurement shown on the pH strip. Similarly, if less than normal levels of acids are being excreted, the pH reading will indicate over-alkalinity.

Since urine pH values can change during the day in reaction to the foods you eat, the best time to measure urine pH is in the morning, soon after you've awakened following at least six hours of sleep, so that your body has had enough time to buffer the effects of your last meal (be sure to avoid eating upon awaking until after you perform this test). The test is easy to perform. Simply take a pH strip and moisten it with your urine as you urinate. A quick dip into your urine stream is all that is necessary. (Be careful not to over-saturate the strip, as doing so can cause a false reading.) As the acid content of your urine reacts with the pH strip, it will change color according to how acidic or alkaline your urine pH is.

Remember, a urine pH test does not provide as accurate an indication of your body's internal acid-alkaline balance, but it can help you get a better sense of the acid or alkaline level in your body. To get a better idea of the state of your body's pH, we recommend that you perform this test every morning for at least one week. If your reading is consistently within the range of 7.0 to 7.5, your body is in a fairly healthy state of acid-alkaline balance. Consistent readings below 7.0 are a good indication that your body is overly acidic.

Interestingly, consistent readings above 7.5 do not necessarily mean your body is overly alkaline. Consistent pH readings above 7.5 can mean one of three things. The first possibility is that your body's internal environment is in a healthy state of acid-alkaline balance or is only slightly alkaline. This is likely to be the case if you regularly consume foods that have an alkalizing effect on the body, and limit your consumption of acid-producing foods, such as meats and dairy products. (More information about both classes of foods is provided in Chapter 4.) Or the reading could be due to supplementing with alkaline mineral supplements for which your body has little use. If any of the above factors apply, a urine pH reading above 7.5 does not indicate imbalance or disease.

Nonetheless, some precautions are advisable. For example, if you are following a vegetarian diet, you should be careful to avoid dietary deficiencies that can be caused by lack of protein from animal products (as well as vitamin deficiencies, such as vitamin B12, which is a common hazard of a strict vegetarian diet). If you are supplementing with alkalizing supplements, it might also be advisable to reduce your intake of them, or to stop taking them altogether.

The second possibility for urine pH readings consistently above 7.5 is far more serious, especially if you are not following an alkalizing diet or taking alkalizing supplements. Such high readings could indicate an imbalance in your endocrine system, which governs the manufacture and regulation of hormones. In particular, a higher pH reading might indicate adrenal or parathyroid gland problems. Or it could be an indication that another form of illness is present. Though such occurrences are rare, it would be wise to consult with your physician to determine if you are at risk for such problems if your pH readings are consistently above 7.5.

In what might seem to be a paradox, the third possibility for

TABLE 3.1 COMMON SYMPTOMS OF ACIDOSIS

CONDITION	SYMPTOMS
Bladder/Urinary	burning sensation during urination, excessive urination, kidney stones
Circulatory Problems	poor circulation, hypotension (low blood pressure), feelings of coldness in the extremities, rapid heartbeat
Energy Levels	chronic fatigue, lack of energy, long recovery time after physical or mental exertion, loss of endurance, easily fatigued after eating meals, chills and/or low body temperature, increased proneness to catch infections
Eye/Facial Problems	conjunctivitis, eyes that tear easily, headache, pale complexion caused by contracting blood vessels
Female Hygiene	vaginal discharge
Gastrointestinal Problems	abdominal pains or cramping, acid reflux, burning sensation in anus or rectum, diarrhea, flatulence, stomach pains or spasms, ulcers
Mental/Emotional Problems	feelings of agitation or nervousness, anxiety, depression, feelings of overwhelm, frequent feelings of stress, irritability, lack of ambition and joy
Mouth and Teeth Problems	bleeding or inflamed gums, cavities, cracked lips, cracked or chipped teeth, loose teeth, mouth ulcers, tooth pain, tooth sensitivity to hot or cold foods
Musculoskeletal Problems	"cracking" joints, muscle cramps or spasms, joint pain, muscle ache, stiff neck, tension in the neck and shoulders
Nail/Hair Problems	brittle or dull hair, hair falling out, thin or splitting nails, white spots or streaks on nails
Respiratory Problems	allergies, chronic bronchitis, frequent colds, frequent coughs or sore throat, laryngitis, runny nose, sensitivity to cold air
Skin Problems	acne, dry skin, eczema, hives, itching, skin blotching or red spots
Sleep Problems	insomnia or restless sleep patterns

consistently high pH readings is that your body is still acidic. If this is the case, it is very likely that you also have difficulty digesting and metabolizing acids. This makes it difficult for your body to oxidize these acids, thus preventing them from being eliminated through respiration. As a result, your kidneys are faced with a greater burden, since more acids are left for them to excrete. Your kidneys can only eliminate a certain amount of acids each day. Once this capacity is met, excess acid stores start to accumulate in your body, forcing it to draw upon its alkaline reserves to neutralize it. Residues of these alkaline minerals get deposited in the urine, thus accounting for the higher pH readings. If this is the case, it is vital that you do all you can to restore your body's internal acid-alkaline balance, because you are most likely on the road to disease.

This third possibility regarding a high urine pH reading is actually fairly common in our society. To help you better determine if you fall into this category, consider whether you are also suffering from and of the symptoms in Table 3.1 (*see* page 51), all of which are common in a state of chronic acidosis. If your are experiencing only one or two such symptoms, your body is not necessarily too acidic, but if more than a few symptoms are present, most likely you fall into this third category.

If you suffer from two or more of these symptoms, there is a high probability that you are also overly acidic, even if your urine pH shows a reading above 7.5. More than likely, you are also eating a diet that is too high in acid-producing foods. As you will learn in Chapter 4, simply changing your diet so that the majority of the foods you eat are alkalizing can make a significant difference in helping to restore your acid-alkaline balance.

Interpreting Your Urine pH Test Results

As you learned in Chapter 1, a pH of 7 is neutral, so any reading below 7 is an acid state and any reading above 7 is an alkaline state. As the body functions best in a slightly alkaline state, for health promotion it is wise to avoid highly acidic metabolic states (or excessive alkaline states, for that matter). Ideally the first morning, the urine reading, after six hours rest, should be between 6.5 and 7.5 on the pH scale, with an occasional, but not regular, higher reading. When your first morning urine is neutral or just slightly acidic, this indicates that your overall cellular pH is approximately alkaline and that the small amounts of acids built up from normal metabolism have been easily concentrated for excretion.

If your pH reading is below 6.5 it is likely that you are experiencing an excessive acid load. This acid load is most likely caused by a diet that is high in acid-forming foods and low in base-forming foods. In this case you would do well to begin making food choice changes aimed at alkalizing your diet. By the way, do not be discouraged if your reading is lower than 6.5. For most Americans this acid tilt is the rule, and the more ideal 6.5 to 7.5 reading the exception. By implementing the information we share in the rest of this book, you can move from acid pH levels to the more ideal slightly alkaline levels fairly easily over a period of a few weeks or months, depending on how out of balance your pH may currently be.

If your urine pH reading is consistently very high (greater than 7.5) this likely indicates a false alkalinity caused by your body being in a catabolic state. This is a state in which the body is breaking down its own tissue. In this breakdown process the amino acid glutamine from the muscles is taken to manufacture ammonia. Ammonia is a strong base that helps the body rid itself of acids when other alkali reserves are depleted. Being a strong base, ammonia alkalizes the urine to an even higher pH level than normally accomplished by alkali mineral salts. This situation of a high "false" alkalinity reflects an underlying acid condition. Alkaline dietary changes are important here also, and in cases of prolonged 7.5 to 8 pH readings it would be wise to consult with a health professional familiar with health restoration and metabolic acidosis.

CONCLUSION

By now you understand why proper acid-alkaline balance is so important to your overall health. You are also now aware of the many symptoms that can occur when this balance is disrupted. In addition, you learned how prolonged pH imbalances can lead to serious health problems, and even prove fatal if they are not addressed in time. Fortunately, as you will see in the following chapters, there is much that you can do on your own to bring your body's pH levels back into balance and, in the process, reverse such problems, starting with your diet.

In the next chapter, you will learn why your diet is so important and how to create a healthy eating plan that supports acid-alkaline imbalance. To learn more, read on.

PART 2

Creating the Acid-Alkaline Lifestyle

4

How Diet Can Restore Acid-Alkaline Balance

A healthy diet is a vital cornerstone of optimal health. As Maimondes, the famed twelfth century physician wrote, "No illness which can be treated by diet should be treated by any other means." This sentiment echoed the instruction expressed by Hippocrates, the Father of Western Medicine, more than a thousand years earlier, when he said, "Let food be thy medicine, and medicine thy food." Such advice goes to the heart of what this book is all about—creating and achieving an acid-alkaline balance.

Why is diet so important to your health? Because the foods you eat supply the fuel your body needs—in the form of vitamins, minerals, enzymes, amino acids, essential fatty acids, and other nutrients—to perform its thousands of daily functions. The better your fuel supply (the foods you eat) is, the better able your body is to generate energy, repair itself, and resist invading pathogens. Conversely, eating poorly diminishes your body's ability to maintain optimum functioning.

Given the important relationship diet has to health, one would think that health experts would agree upon what constitutes a healthy diet. Unfortunately, one of the public's leading complaints relates to their confusion over the vast amount of conflicting nutritional advice provided by today's so-called health experts. This is due, in no small part, to the many books on the subject that are published each year touting the "latest and greatest" cure-all diet. Simply check the current list of nonfiction bestsellers for the "breakthrough" diet books—from low-fat to no-fat and from low carbs to high proteins. Because of how contradictory these books can be to each other, it is no wonder that so many of us say they are literally "fed up" with dietary advice.

Eating healthy should not be an exercise in fads or pot luck. And it does not have to be, as you will soon discover in the pages ahead. The key to eating well is to eat foods that will provide your body with what it needs to maintain a healthy pH. In this chapter we will show you how to do so easily and without confusion. First, let's examine some important general guidelines for eating healthy.

HEALTHY EATING BASICS

The following healthy eating guidelines have long been recommended by nutritionally oriented physicians and many health organizations, yet they continued to be ignored by tens of millions of Americans, a fact that goes a long way toward explaining our nation's current healthcare crisis. Given that healthy diet alone can greatly reduce your risk of serious health conditions, including our nation's two top killers—heart disease and cancer—we cannot emphasize enough how important these guidelines can be to your health.

Eat fresh fruits and vegetables. A plentiful supply of fresh fruits and vegetables should be a daily staple of your diet. Both of these food groups are rich with vital nutrients and enzymes, and also high in fiber. Be sure to eat at least a portion of your daily vegetable intake raw, since high temperatures from cooking can destroy their nutrient and enzyme content. (More information on the merits of eating raw versus cooked vegetables is provided on page 77.) Lightly steaming vegetables is another healthy cooking alternative.

Eat a variety of foods. Many people today are deficient in essential nutrients because they routinely eat a limited variety of foods meal after meal. Not only does such "diet monotony" limit nutrient intake, it also can lead to food allergies and sensitivities, both of which are common, yet frequently undiagnosed health conditions. By eating a wide variety of foods, you have a much better likelihood of avoiding such conditions, and can also increase your nutrient intake.

Eat organic foods. Whenever possible, we recommend that you eat organic foods. Organic fruits and vegetables have been shown to have a higher nutrient content, compared to non-organic produce, and are also free of harmful pesticides, preservatives, and other chemicals used to grow non-organic, commercial food crops. Similarly, your meat and poultry food choices should ideally be free-range and free of the hormones and antibiotics that are commonly given to commercially harvested animal products.

Maximize your intake of essential fatty acids. Contrary to popular belief, all of us require a certain amount of fat in our diet. Fats act as the bodies' energy reserves, and serve as a primary form of insulation, helping to maintain normal body temperature. In addition, fats assist in transporting oxygen, help in the absorption of fat-soluble vitamins, and act as natural anti-inflammatory agents. Fats also help nourish the skin, nerves, and mucous membranes. The best sources of fat in the diet are essential fatty acids (EFAs), particularly omega-3s and omega-6s. Many people have an excess of omega-6s in their diet, compared to omega-3s, so taking care to ensure a proper balance between the two is important. Good sources of omega-3 EFAs include herring, mackerel, sardines, wild-caught salmon, wild game, flaxseed and flaxseed oil, walnuts, and pumpkin seeds.

Eat plenty of fiber. The standard American diet supplies no more than a third (and often even less) of the amount of fiber necessary for optimum health. Yet research shows that a high fiber diet is closely associated with lower incidences of heart disease, high blood pressure, certain types of cancer (especially colon and rectal cancer), diabetes, constipation, hemorrhoids, gall bladder disease, and gastrointestinal conditions such as colitis and diverticulitis. Good sources of fiber include fruits, vegetables, bran, rolled oats, brown rice, and other complex carbohydrates.

Eliminate "junk" foods. Simply put, junk foods are unhealthy and, when eaten on a regular basis, will inevitably lead to disease. These foods are so named because they are overloaded with chemicals, colorings, trans-fats, excess sugars, and other additives that are bad for our health. Moreover, they are typically high in calories and low in nutrient content, and are among the leading causes of acid-alkaline imbalance. If you truly are committed to your health, you will avoid eating such foods altogether.

Eliminate simple sugars and refined carbohydrates. The average American consumes 150 pounds of simple or refined sugar each and every year. This is the equivalent of more than 40 teaspoons of sugar a day, which goes a long way towards explaining why, as a nation, we are so sick. Sugar's many harmful effects include increasing the risk of heart disease, weakening the immune system and increasing susceptibility to infection, stimulating excessive insulin production, increasing the production of harmful triglycerides, diminishing mental function, increasing feelings of anxiety and depression, increasing the risk of cancer, and increasing systemic yeast overgrowth (candidiasis). To effectively eliminate sugar from your diet, it is important that you read food labels, since sugar is a common ingredient in packaged foods in the forms of fructose, sucrose, corn syrup, lactose, and maltose. In general, foods that are frozen, canned, processed, or cured are also likely to be high in sugar. Healthy sugar substitutes include raw, organic honey, stevia, and, eaten sparingly, dark chocolate.

Refined carbohydrates essentially act in much the same way that sugar does when consumed and metabolized in your body. Therefore, they should be avoided altogether.

Refined, or simple, carbohydrates, such as white breads, pastas made from white flour, instant mashed potatoes, white rice, chips, and sugar laden commercial cereals, are another unfortunate staple of the "standard American diet" and pose additional health risks. The most common health risks when these foods are consumed on a regular basis are excessive insulin production, excessive fat storage, and elevated blood sugar levels. Obesity and diabetes are two of the most serious health conditions directly linked to frequent consumption of these foods.

Eliminate unhealthy fats. As previously mentioned, certain fats are essential for good health. Unfortunately, many of us, instead of eating foods rich in healthy fats, consume harmful fats such as trans-fatty acids and hydrogenated fats, both of which have been linked to a host of disease conditions, including arteriosclerosis, heart attack, angina, cancer, kidney failure, and obesity. Trans-fatty acids and hydrogenated fats are commonly found in margarine, cooking fats, commercial peanut butter, commercial cereals, and packaged foods.

Have some saturated fat—contrary to popular belief, it's good for you. Until recently, saturated fats, found in red meats, milk, butter, cheese and other dairy products, were also linked to health problems, and recommended to be consumed sparingly. New evidence, however, suggests that the health risks of saturated fat consumption have been overstated, and that moderate saturated fat consumption is actually good for you. So don't worry about treating yourself to such foods, just take care not to overdo it.

Minimize caffeine. It is estimated that more than half of all Americans are addicted to caffeine, primarily through drinking coffee. While caffeine in moderation (one to two cups of coffee per day) is not only harmless, but provides a variety of health benefits, too much regular caffeine consumption can contribute to a wide range of health problems, and can decrease platelet stickiness, thus interfering with the blood clotting process. It can also cause loss of calcium in the body, thereby disrupting the acid-alkaline balance. If you enjoy drinking coffee, we recommend organic blends.

Minimize, don't eliminate your salt intake. Salt is another ingredient that is far too prevalent in the standard American diet. However, a certain amount of salt is required by your body in order to carry out its many functions. It's when we consume too much salt that health problems can arise. When salt intake is excessive, water is drawn into the bloodstream, increasing blood volume. This, in turn, can increase blood pressure levels, and also interfere with the ability of the body's lymphatic system to eliminate waste matter from the cells.

Additionally, many brands of commercial salt are devoid of iodine (which is essential for proper thyroid function) and other essential trace minerals that are found in salt in its natural state. Therefore, we recommend that, when you do use salt, you choose sea or Celtic salt, both of which are rich in such co-factor minerals.

Drink alcohol only in moderation. Although in recent years a number of studies have indicated that consumption of wine or beer in moderation may provide health benefits, such as reduced stress and improved digestion, for many people, alcohol and moderation don't always go together well. In addition to the well-known social problems associated with alcohol abuse, too much alcohol has been directly linked to a variety of disease conditions, including hypertension, diabetes, obesity, gastrointestinal disorders, impaired liver function, candidiasis, cancer, impaired mental function, and behavioral and emotional problems. Moreover, although many people drink in order to feel better, research conducted by the National Center for Health Statistics found that alcohol consumption can result in pronounced feelings of loneliness and depression.

Alcoholic beverages for which health benefits have been shown are beer and wine, especially red wine. For men, one or two glasses of beer or wine per day is permissible, while women should limit their intake of these beverages to one glass per day. "Hard" alcohol, such as whiskey, bourbon, brandy, and others should be avoided altogether.

By following the above guidelines, you can improve your health over time. The key is to commit yourself to making them a regular part of your daily life. Now let's explore how you can improve these guidelines even further by eating to achieve and maintain acid-alkaline balance, which will enable you to far more quickly progress down the road to lasting health and vitality.

HOW THE FOODS YOU EAT EFFECT YOUR BODY'S ACID-ALKALINE BALANCE

As we discussed earlier, all of the foods you eat, once they are digested and metabolized (literally burned down), leave a residue of food ash in your body. Depending on the type of food you eat and its mineral content, the ash residue is acidic, alkaline, or neutral. Foods that produce an acidic ash residue have an acidifying effect on the body and lower pH levels. Foods that leave an alkaline effect have the opposite effect, being alkalizing and raising pH levels. Foods that produce a neutral ash residue have little to no effect on pH levels. Generally speaking, foods eaten raw tend to also produce an alkalizing effect on pH levels, compared to cooked foods, which typically are acidifying in nature.

It is important to note that the acidifying, alkalizing, or neutral effects produced by the foods you eat are far more significant, in terms of your health, than the foods' inherent pH values prior to their consumption. For example, a number of foods that are acidic in nature, such as certain citrus fruits and vinegars, actually produce an alkalizing effect on the body after they are digested and metabolized. Not all acidic foods are acidifying when eaten, nor are all alkaline foods alkalizing when consumed. Therefore, knowing the effect a food will have on your pH levels is the key to choosing your foods wisely.

Ironically, the acidifying and alkalizing effects of foods are too often ignored by dieticians and nutritionists who focus solely on foods' nutrient content. Nutrients are, of course, essential to good health. But when pH levels are imbalanced, proper absorption and utilization of nutrients is interrupted, eventually resulting in nutritional deficiencies. Fortunately, by following the guidelines in this chapter, you will be able to achieve optimal pH levels and obtain all the nutrients your body needs—properly delivered to your cells and tissues.

Before listing the most common acidifying and alkalizing foods, here are some guidelines that will help you make your food selections.

- In general, your diet should be comprised of between 60 to 80 percent of foods that are alkalizing. If your pH levels are more than slightly acidic, then alkalizing foods should comprise approximately 80 percent of your daily dietary intake. A basic rule of thumb to remember is this: *The more you suffer from over-acidity, the more alkalizing foods you should consume.*

- It is also important to eat more alkalizing foods at every meal, rather than eating all your alkalizing foods at one or two meals, and eating acidifying foods the rest of the day. This absolutely includes snacks. And never try to eat meals consisting solely of acidifying foods, such as pasta with meatballs or steak and potatoes.

- By eating a higher proportion of alkalizing foods at every meal, your body will become better able to neutralize whatever acids are produced during digestion. Eating this way will safeguard your body from the burden of further acidity. It will also allow your body's detoxification system to more effectively reduce and eliminate toxic acids that have already built up inside of you.

- If you are like most people, you may need to eat greater amounts of alkalizing foods initially. But over time, as your pH levels become more balanced, you will be able to make adjustments to your diet. You will be able to lower the amounts (60 percent) of alkalizing foods you eat, and still maintain the improvements to your health. Once you achieve and stabilize your ideal pH level, you may even find you can eat equal amounts of alkalizing and acidifying foods without any problems. Overall, however, we recommend that you continue to eat a higher proportion of alkalizing foods than foods that produce acidic effects, even after your health and energy levels return to normal.

- Since alkalizing foods play a significant role in helping to bring overly acidic pH levels back into balance, you may think it wise to drastically reduce your intake of acidifying foods, or to eliminate them altogether. *Don't!* No matter how acidic your pH may be, your body still requires foods that are rich in proteins in order to function properly. Foods with the highest concentration of proteins are meats, fish, eggs, milk, and dairy products, all of which produce highly acidifying effects in the body. But if you eliminate such foods from your diet altogether, you will not be able to achieve acid-alkaline balance.

- In order for your body to function it requires a certain amount of acidifying protein for it to establish alkaline minerals in your tissues. It is protein that enables your tissues to retain these alkaline minerals. By eliminating protein, you eliminate some of these minerals that protect you when harmful acids need to be neutralized. When this occurs, the acids spread throughout your body, forcing it to call on stored mineral reserves, eventually to the point where those reserves are completely depleted. The end result is greater acidity and the onset of the diseases it can cause.

- There may be times when an all-alkaline diet is warranted, such as in cases of pronounced acidosis, accompanied by painful symptoms. But such a diet should only be in use for a short duration—no more than one or two weeks. By following an entirely alkaline diet of vegetables and fruits, the body would have a chance to recover more rapidly. But to continue on such a diet once symptoms abate would not be wise due to its lack of protein and various nutrients.

The exception to the above guidelines is for people whose pH levels are overly alkaline. Admittedly, such people are rare, given the highly acidifying effects of the standard American diet, but if you fall into this category, you will want to increase your intake of acidifying foods until your pH returns to normal. After that, you will want to monitor your pH and follow the guidelines above. (*See* Table 4.1 below for more specific guidelines.)

TABLE 4.1. ACID-ALKALINE DIET EATING PLANS		
	ACID-TO-ALKALINE FOOD PERCENTAGE	
PH LEVEL	ACID FOODS	ALKALINE FOODS
Too Alkaline	20 to 40 percent	60 to 80 percent
Normal	50 percent	50 percent
Too Acidic	20 percent	80 percent
Extremely Acidic	100 percent	

(The diet of 100 percent alkalizing foods should be followed for one to two weeks only, after which the "Too Acidic" diet should be followed.)

ACIDIFYING AND ALKALIZING FOODS

As we've discussed, the foods we eat can be divided into three distinct categories in terms of how they affect pH levels: acidifying, alkalizing, and neutral. However, it is also important to know the degree to which foods produce their effects. For example, grains such as brown rice and millet both produce an acidifying effect in the body when they are eaten, but brown rice is far less acidifying than millet.

Compounding this issue is the fact that your unique biochemistry brings with it its own inherent strengths and weakness with regard to how the foods you eat will affect you. As you begin to adopt the specific eating plan we are recommending, pay careful attention to how you feel following each meal. A food that produces only a mild acidifying effect for most people might produce a very acidifying effect for you. Should this occur, trust your own experience, and adapt accordingly. In general, however, the classification of food groups that follow—further subdivided into categories of very acidifying, mildly acidifying, very alkalizing, mildly alkalizing, and neutral—is accurate for the vast majority of people.

Acidifying Foods

Acidifying foods are generally high in proteins, carbohydrates, and/or fats. Such foods include:

- alcohol
- breads
- caffeine products, (chocolate, coffee, black tea)
- commercial condiments
- fish
- certain grains
- legumes
- meats
- milk and dairy products
- poultry
- refined and processed foods
- seeds and nuts
- Soda
- sugars and artificial sweeteners
- tap water
- yeast products

Alcohol. All forms of alcoholic beverages cause acidification in the body. One of the by-products of alcohol when it is metabolized in the body is acetaldehyde. This is a compound that acts as a toxin in the body. While recent research indicates that moderate consumption of beer or wine can enhance health by relieving stress and improving digestion, we recommend that when you drink such beverages that you accompany them with a glass of water to minimize their acidifying effects.

Artificial sweeteners. Many people who seek to eliminate sugar from their diet choose to use artificial sweeteners as substitutes under the mistaken belief that they are healthier. Nothing could be further from the truth. Products, such as aspartame (NutraSweet), saccharine, and cyclamates, are extremely acidifying. In addition, a number of the chemical ingredients they contain have been linked to a wide range of disease conditions and symptoms. If you are seeking a healthy substitute for artificial sweeteners, we recommend stevia or xylitol.

Breads. All breads create an acidifying effect in the body. Some breads however are more acidifying than others. Whole grain breads are less acidifying than refined white breads, for example, as are yeast-free breads compared to breads containing yeast. As a rule, you should eat bread sparingly, if at all, and avoid white breads and breads made from yeast entirely. If you choose to eat bread, you can reduce its acidifying effects by toasting it first.

Caffeine products. Foods in this group include chocolate, cocoa, teas, and all forms of coffee, including decaffeinated coffees. Caffeine produces high amounts of acidic residues in the body, and is also mucus forming. More than 50 percent of all Americans are estimated to be addicted to caffeine, primarily in the form of coffee, which they consume throughout the day in order to have energy. Ironically, caffeine actually drains the body's energy reserves, creating a harmful cycle where caffeine drinkers need another drink of coffee as soon as the artificial energy jolt from their last cup wears off.

Commercial condiments. The primary offenders in this category are mayonnaise, ketchup, and mustard, all prized staples of the standard American diet. Most of the commercial products available also contain sugar, as well as other unhealthy additives. If you don't wish to eliminate these products completely, at least use them sparingly, and choose brands that are organic. Or, better yet, consider using healthy substitutes, such as natural herbs and spices, sea salt, or kelp, to add flavor to the dishes you prepare. (*See* Herbs, Spices, and Salts on page 79.)

Commercial juices and sports drinks. Beverages in this category include commercial fruit and vegetable juices and sports drinks such as Gatorade and Red Bull. Commercial fruit and vegetable juices are largely devoid of nutrients, which are destroyed in their manufacturing process, and therefore provide little health benefit. In addition, commercial juices can be acidifying, and vegetable brands also contain harmful additives, such as high amounts of salt (sodium). They are no substitute for freshly squeezed juices which you can easily make at home should you care to invest in a home juicer. Not only will such homemade juices provide you with a rich supply of important vitamin, minerals, and other nutrients, they are also very alkalizing.

Sports drinks are highly acidifying, which is not surprising, since sugar, in the form of fructose or other sugar compounds, is one of their principal ingredients. So-called energy drinks such as Red Bull also contain high amounts of caffeine. We recommend that you avoid both classes of beverages altogether.

Fish, meats, and poultry. All meats and meat by-products, including animal fats, create an acidifying effect in the body because of their high protein content. After such foods are digested and metabolized, they leave behind residues of uric acid. This can cause toxic acid buildup in the body. Meats also contain phosphorus and sulfur, two minerals that also are acidifying. In addition, commercially harvested meats, fish, and poultry are usually laced with hormones, pesticides, steroids, and antibiotics, all of which are very harmful to your health.

Animal fats—often used in cooking and deep-frying—contribute to acidic pH because they are high in saturated fatty acids. These fats are difficult for the body to properly digest and metabolize. Incomplete digestion of saturated fatty acids results in the creation of toxic waste products that place a further burden on the body's ability to maintain balanced acid-alkaline levels. Given the high fat content of the standard American diet, it is little wonder that acidification due to unhealthy fat consumption is quite common in the United States.

A certain amount of fish, meats, and poultry can be very beneficial for your health, however, especially fish that is wild-caught as opposed to farm raised, and grass-fed meats and free-range poultry. As we explained in Chapter 1, protein intake up to 50 to 63 grams a day, when eaten with a variety of alkalizing foods, will not create an acidic debt in the bodies of most people, since the alkalizing foods will neutralize the acidic ash created when protein foods are digested and metabolized. As with many other health related issues, when it comes to fish, meats, and poultry, moderation is the key.

Grains. Both whole and refined grains are for the most part acidifying. This includes rice, oats, wheat, and millet. Grains are primarily composed of carbohydrates, which are often poorly digested due to the fact that many people unknowingly are sensitive or allergic to them. Interestingly, however, when grains are sprouted, they become alkalizing foods, and have the same positive effects on the body as do green vegetables. For this reason, we recommend that you consider making sprouted grain products a staple of your diet, while using non-sprouted grains sparingly. (*See* page 000 for more information about sprouts.)

Legumes. Legumes are a class of vegetables consisting of beans and peas that contain edible seeds inside their pods. Foods in the legumes group include aduki beans, black beans, black-eyed peas, chickpeas, great northern beans, green beans, green peas, kidney beans, lentils, lima beans, mung beans, navy beans, pinto beans, and soybeans. Legumes are low in calories and provide a nice balance of proteins and complex carbohydrates. They are also a staple food for many people around the world because of their nutritious value.

Legumes can also create acidic conditions in the body, however. The most acidifying foods in this category include peanuts, chickpeas, peas, and most beans, including soybeans. Peanut products, such as peanut butter, also fall into this category. When such foods are digested and metabolized, they leave behind a residue of uric acid that can contribute to acidosis. Because of their nutritious qualities, we do not recommend that you completely eliminate legumes from your diet. Rather, feel free to include them in your meal plans, but do so in moderation. To further enhance the nutritious benefits they provide, also consider sprouting them (for more on sprouts and sprouting, *see* page 80). Not only does sprouting dramatically reduce legumes' acidifying effects, it also increases their nutritional value.

Milk and dairy products. Included in this group are butter, cheese, eggs and yogurt. Cheeses with a sharp flavor, such as cheddar, are more acidifying than milder, white cheeses. In addition to causing acidification, milk and dairy products contain casein which produces mucus buildup.

Many people are also unknowingly allergic or sensitive to milk and dairy products due to their inability to tolerate lactose, a form of sugar contained in such foods. Unfortunately, commercial milk also contains a multitude of chemicals fed to cows that have been found to be unhealthy to humans. This includes hormones, antibiotics, pesticides, as well as hundreds of other substances used to increase milk production.

Organic versions of these foods are your best choices when it comes to your health, but even they should be consumed in moderation. An exception to this rule is eggs. Once demonized as an unhealthy food, researchers now recognize eggs as one of nature's healthiest foods. One or two eggs per day is perfectly acceptable for most people, but, again, choose organic brands. Additionally, if you enjoy milk, consider milk alternatives such as almond or coconut milk, both of which are slightly alkalizing.

Refined and processed foods. Foods in this category include fast foods, candies, donuts and pastries, refined flour and breads, refined grain products (including white flour pastas), and commercial cereals. Not only are such foods in this category highly acidifying, they have also been stripped of essential nutrients through the refinement process. In addition, they contain artificial chemical flavorings, colorings, and preservatives that are completely foreign to the body's digestive system. They are also high in sugars and hydrogenated or partially hydrogenated oils, all of which act as poisons in the body and have been linked to degenerative disease, including cancer. Regular consumption of such foods is a sure recipe for major health problems. They should be eliminated completely from your diet.

Seeds and nuts. With certain exceptions, such as almonds and Brazil nuts (*see* page 79 for more information on these nuts), nearly all seeds and nuts lower pH values in the body, creating acidity. Foods in this category include pumpkin, sesame, and sunflower seeds, as well as cashews, hazelnuts, pecans, and walnuts. All of these foods contain phosphorous and sulfur, and are high in fats, all of which can contribute to acidification. Since seeds and nuts are also rich in other nutrients, however, we are in favor of making them part of your regular food intake, so long as they are eaten in moderation. By soaking seeds and nuts overnight, you can further minimize their acidic effects.

Soda. Soda is one of the most highly acidifying substances you can consume, especially the colas. Not only do sodas have high sugar content, they also contain high levels of caffeine, further adding to the problem.

To give you a better idea of how toxic the effects of soda are on your body, consider this finding from researcher Sang Wang, author of the book *Reverse Aging:* In order to neutralize a glass of soda, 32 glasses of highly alkaline water are required. We recommend that you eliminate soda altogether. As a substitute, you may use unflavored seltzer water or club soda, but we recommend that you do so sparingly.

Sugar. Sugar is seemingly everywhere in the standard American diet. It can be found under the following names: white sugar, brown sugar, cane sugar, corn sugar, date sugar, fructose, galactose, glucose, lactose, maltose, mannitol, and sorbitol. Honey, maple syrup, and molasses are other sugar-rich foods.

Commercial white sugar, a staple, for example, of jellies, candies, and pastries, is also refined, meaning it contains no vitamins, minerals, or enzymes. The absence of such nutrients makes it extremely difficult for the body to metabolize sugar. Sugar also forces the body to release stored vitamins and minerals in an attempt to convert it to energy. This, in turn, reduces the available supply of stored nutrients that the body would otherwise need to function properly, including maintaining homeostasis and balanced pH levels.

Sugar also poses other serious health risks. It is one of the primary substances used by cancer cells to fuel their growth and proliferation. It acts as fuel for harmful microorganisms in the body. As these microorganisms die and decompose, the fermentation they cause increases the body's acidity, creating additional health burdens. For all of these reasons, we recommend that you completely eliminate added sugars from your diet. Foods containing naturally-occurring sugars, especially fruits, are permissible, but should be eaten sparingly, with the exception of lemons, limes, and avocados, due to their highly alkalizing effects.

Tap water. Unlike pure, filtered water, which is either pH-neutral or has a slightly alkalizing effect when consumed, tap water is not only acidifying but most likely contains both fluoride and chlorine, both of which have been linked to cancer and a variety of other degenerative diseases. Most municipal tap water supplies in the United States also contain a cocktail of other harmful metals and other additives and, as a result of the widespread use of pharmaceutical drugs across our nation, pharmaceutical drug residues caused by such drugs finding their way into our water supplies after being flushed down the toilet. All of these contaminants are not only highly acidifying, they are also highly toxic.

For these reasons, we recommend that you avoid using tap water altogether, even when steaming vegetables. This includes bathing and showering in tap water, since the harmful chemicals it contains are also absorbed through the skin. You can reduce this problem significantly by investing in water filters for your faucet and showerhead. Just be sure to change the filter cartridges according to directions.

To avoid drinking tap water, bottled water has become increasingly popular in this country. We don't agree with this trend for a number of reasons.

- First, lab tests show that many brands of bottled water are no safer, and in some cases even more unsafe, than tap water.

- Second, the cost of bottled water is actually very expensive, given how little it costs the bottled water industry to package and supply it.

- Third, unless you are buying water in glass bottles, the far more prevalent plastic bottles it comes in very likely contains harmful chemicals, such as bisphenol A (BPA), a chemical that can leach into the water before it is consumed, and which has been linked to a variety of health problems ranging from endocrine disruption to behavioral problems (especially among babies and children) to brain disorders.

- Finally, the increased use of bottled water in the US has created a dramatic swell in the amount of plastic bottles in our nation's landfills, and also in many lakes, riverbeds, and even the ocean due to how frequently such bottles are cast aside as litter. If you wish to continue to drink bottled water, we highly recommend that you purchase a reusable, non-plastic water bottle that you can fill and carry with you when you leave your home.

Yeast products. Besides brewer's and baker's yeast, yeast products include breads and baked goods, beer, and wine. Yeast is also often an ingredient in commercial condiments and seasonings.

Yeast consumption can also promote the proliferation of *Candida albicans,* the microorganism responsible for candidiasis, or systemic yeast overgrowth in the body. Candidiasis is a widespread problem among many people suffering from chronic health problems such as allergies, anxiety and depression, chronic fatigue, fungal infections, gastrointestinal disorders, memory problems, mood swings, respiratory problems, and sleep disturbances. All yeast products are acidifying, and should therefore be used sparingly, if at all.

Aside from those products that we indicated should be completely eliminated, the foods and beverages discussed above can still remain a part of your dietary intake. But you should consume them sparingly, limiting their combined intake to no more than 40 percent of the foods and beverages you consume each day, and ideally reducing them down to 20 percent, especially if you are already suffering from chronic health problems. And always remember to eat a greater supply of alkalizing foods alongside of them at every meal to help neutralize their acidifying effects.

Alkalizing Foods

Alkalizing foods are rich in alkaline minerals and contain little to no acidic substances. In addition, these foods produce no acidic ash when they are digested and metabolized, regardless of how much of them are consumed at any meal. Foods in this category include all green vegetables, most colored vegetables, cold-pressed oils, sprouts, certain fruits and nuts, herbs and spices, and alkaline mineral water. Everyone suffering from chronic acidosis needs to include these foods at every meal, in much greater proportions (as high as 80 percent) than acidifying foods eaten at the same time.

Alkaline mineral water. Water in its natural state normally has a neutral pH of 7.0. Most tap water has an acidic pH, however. This is due to chlorination and fluoridation. The same is true of carbonated water. Many brands of mineral water, on the other hand, are alkalizing because of the alkaline minerals they contain. Such brands also list their pH values right on the label, making it easy for you to determine their degree of alkalinity.

Cold-pressed oils. Cold-pressed oils are oils that are prepared without using heat or chemicals when they are extracted from their food sources (borage, flax seed, hemp seed, and olives). Commercial methods of oils extraction not only destroy at least part of the oils' nutrient supply, they also cause the oils to breakdown during processing, making them harder for your body to digest and metabolize. Cold-pressed oils are an important source of essential fatty acids (EFAs).

EFAs are monounsaturated or polyunsaturated fats that are converted by the body into hormone-like substances known as prostaglandins, which regulate the body's inflammatory response, and nourish body fats used to strengthen cell walls and provide cellular energy. EFAs also play an important role in strengthening the immune system. The EFAs contained in cold-pressed oils also help to bind and eliminate acids in the body. Good sources of cold-pressed oils include borage, evening primrose, flax, and olive oil. Of these, only olive oil should be used for cooking. Flaxseed oil can be added to foods after they have been prepared, and can be a delicious complement to salads because of its rich, nutty flavor. Borage and evening primrose oils are primarily used as nutritional supplements because of their value as sources of EFAs.

Another versatile and healthy oil with alkalizing benefits is coconut oil. It, too, is an excellent oil for cooking. In addition, research shows that coconut oil offers a variety of other important health benefits, including as a brain food that can help prevent the onset of dementia and Alzheimer's disease. Coconut oil also has strong anti-viral and anti-bacterial properties. Taking one or two tablespoons of coconut oil per day is therefore a good idea as part of your overall health maintenance program, especially during cold and flu season. For best results when using any of the above oils choose brands that are certified organic.

Fruits. Though fruits are rich in essential nutrients, enzymes, and fiber, they are also abundant in natural sugars. This makes most fruits slightly acidifying when they are eaten. Most people should eat such fruits sparingly.

The exceptions to this rule are bananas, grapefruit, lemons, limes, avocados, and tomatoes. (Though avocados and tomatoes are often considered to be vegetables, in actuality they are fruits. They are most alkalizing when eaten raw.) Bananas are naturally alkaline, whereas grapefruit, lemons and limes are acidic in nature. However, during the digestive process, as grapefruit, lemons, and limes are metabolized, they produce a highly alkalizing effect. All three of these fruits are also naturally rich in oxygen, further aiding their alkalizing abilities.

An easy and effective way to help your body maintain proper acid-alkaline balance is to begin each day with a glass of purified water combined with fresh squeezed lemon juice. Or, if you prefer, you can substitute lime. (Make sure you use organic fruits whenever possible.) This serves as an excellent tonic to get your morning started, and is highly alkalizing. Wait 20 to 30 minutes before you eat anything, to gain the full benefits.

Dried fruits, including dates, also produce an alkalizing effect in the body. This occurs because their acid content is oxidized during the drying process. To get the most benefits from eating dried fruit, be sure to select ones that are free of sulfur, which is often used as a preservative in commercial brands. Since dried fruits also have a high natural sugar content, they should be eaten sparingly.

Green and colored vegetables. The foundation of every alkalizing meal is plenty of vegetables, which should always be included as part of your lunch and dinner. Raw vegetables such as celery also make an ideal snack food during the day. Servings of green vegetables throughout the day are particularly potent aids in restoring acid-alkaline balance.

All vegetables are rich in vitamins, alkalizing minerals and salts, enzymes, phytonutrients (nutrients derived from plant foods), and fiber. But green vegetables are also rich in chlorophyll, which is what gives them their green color. Chlorophyll contains many of the same chemical components as hemoglobin. Leafy green vegetables are particularly rich sources of chlorophyll. (For more on chlorophyll, *see* The Relationship Between Blood and Chlorophyll on page 78.)

Don't neglect other colored vegetables, though. While not as rich in chlorophyll, they too are excellent sources of essential nutrients. Vegetables in this category that you can eat freely include beets, yellow cabbage, carrots, cauliflower, garlic, onions, potatoes, radishes, red and yellow peppers, scallions, turnips, and yellow squash.

Ideally, you should eat a certain amount of raw vegetables every day, while lightly steaming or sautéing the rest. This will ensure that the rich supply of enzymes, vegetables contain, are not destroyed by overcooking. Enzymes are contained in all fresh fruits and vegetables and play an essential role in healthy digestion. When enzymes are deficient in your diet, your body is unable to properly digest and assimilate the foods you eat, setting the stage for further health problems. Enzymes are inactivated and destroyed when vegetables are cooked in temperatures over 118 degrees. (For more on enzymes, *see* page 124.)

Whenever possible, it is also a good idea to select organically grown vegetables, which contain more abundant amounts of essential nutrients than do commercially grown produce, and are also free of pesticides and other harmful chemicals. Organic vegetables are now readily available in health food stores and commercial chain grocery food stores. You can also find them at your local farm stands and farmers' markets. Whether you use organic or non-organic produce, always be sure to wash them thoroughly.

The Relationship Between Blood and Chlorophyll

One of the primary benefits of regularly consuming green vegetables is the supply of chlorophyll you will receive as a result. Chlorophyll is often referred to as the "blood" of vegetables, with good reason. Chlorophyll's chemical makeup and molecular structure is closely related to hemoglobin, a prime component of human blood.

Hemoglobin is rich in iron, and plays an important role in delivering oxygen to your body's cells and tissues. In addition to iron, hemoglobin is composed of carbon, hydrogen, oxygen, and nitrogen. In comparison, chlorophyll is made up of the very same elements, except that it contains magnesium instead of iron.

The more green, chlorophyll-rich vegetables you consume each day, the more you will enhance your body's ability to transport oxygen to all of your cells and tissues, for this is exactly what chlorophyll does once the green vegetables you eat are digested and metabolized. Chlorophyll also helps the liver and other organs detoxify, and it prevents carcinogens (cancer-causing toxins) from binding to cellular DNA. It aids in the breakdown and elimination of calcium stones, as well. This is of particular importance to people who are chronically overly acidic, since calcium stones are one of the ways the body attempts to neutralize excess acid buildup. With all of these health-producing benefits, you can clearly see why we recommend that you make green vegetables an important part of your daily dietary intake.

And if you suffer from sugar sensitivities and/or are hyper- or hypoglycemic, initially you may want to avoid or minimize eating vegetables that have a naturally high sugar content, such as beets, carrots, and squash. Over time, however, as your health improves and your sugar problems stabilize, these vegetables can be added back to your diet and eaten in moderation.

Herbs, spices, and salts. Herbs and spices have been used for centuries for their health-promoting properties. Most herbs and spices have an alkalizing effect on the body, as well. This includes herbal teas. Certain herbs, such as cayenne pepper, cinnamon, garlic, oregano, and sage, also function as spices that can add flavor to your meals. Unlike processed table salt, which should be avoided due to its acidifying effects, unprocessed sea salt and Celtic salt can also be used to spice up your meals. Both forms of these salts are alkalizing and are also rich in iodine, which is essential for healthy thyroid function.

Nuts and seeds. A variety of nuts and seeds are also alkalizing. Among the most alkalizing nuts are almonds, Brazil nuts, cashews, chestnuts, and macadamia nuts. Brazil nuts are also a rich source of the trace mineral selenium, which is often lacking in the standard American diet, and which has been shown to have anti-cancer properties. Almond milk, made by combining purified water with almond paste, is an excellent alternative to dairy and soymilk because of its alkalizing effects.

Alkalizing seeds include celery seeds, cumin seeds, flaxseed, hemp seeds, pumpkin seeds, and sunflower seeds. All such seeds make a healthy addition to salads.

Both nuts and seeds are also packed with many important nutrients, making them an ideal choice for healthy snacks during the day. However, because of their high caloric content, nuts and seeds should be eaten sparingly, usually no more than one or two handfuls at a time.

Potatoes. Potatoes are another class of alkalizing vegetables. Historically, potatoes have been a staple food in every culture in which they are indigenous. But with all the emphasis today on "low-carb" diets, many people are eliminating potatoes from their diets. For people who need to shift their pH levels to a more alkaline state, neglecting potatoes can be a big mistake.

Unlike cereals and grains, which for the most part have an acidifying effect on the body, potatoes are very high in alkalizing nutrients. In fact, because of its alkalizing effects, many native healers and naturopathic physicians often recommend potato juice as a first resort for relieving ulcers and stomach problems caused by over-acidity. Potato skins are also a rich source of vitamin C, and potatoes can help fuel your body's energy supply, as well.

Unfortunately, in today's standard American diet, the health-giving properties in potatoes are often destroyed because of the way they are prepared or served. Even when they are not transformed into French fries, an extremely acidic junk-food, they are often buried beneath heaps of sour cream, another acidifying substance. By contrast, baked or boiled potatoes, served with a small dollop of organic butter or cold-pressed olive oil, along with a dash of herbs or spices, makes for a nutritious side-dish packed with potent alkalizing benefits. Or, if you prefer, you can choose to eat yams, the potato's more colorful cousin, which provide similar benefits.

Sprouts. Sprouts are a special class of food produced from the germination of beans, grains, and seeds. The germination process requires no soil, only water and a cool room temperature. In the sprouting process even foods that in their normal state are acidifying, such as beans and grains. They become alkalizing due to what happens to them as they are sprouted. For example, proteins, fats, and starches are transformed into more easily digestible and assimilated amino acids, fatty acids, and vegetable sugars. In addition, sprouting also increases the amounts of certain nutrients sprouted foods contain, especially the B vitamins, which can increase from 50 to over 1,000 percent after beans, grains, and seeds are sprouted. Sprouts are also energy-rich foods that are high in enzymes, proteins, vitamins, minerals, and other vital nutrients.

How to Make Your Own Sprouts

Sprouting beans, grains, and seeds is very easy to do. All that is required are the foods themselves, purified water, and a glass quart jar with a mesh top held in place by rubber bands. To begin, select the type of foods you wish to sprout and soak them overnight in purified water. The next morning, drain and place them in the jar, then place the jar in a warm, dry area. Twice a day, rinse the contents (pouring the water out through the mesh covering when you are done).

Depending on the bean, grain, or seed you choose (whenever possible, make sure they are organic), your sprouts will be ready for eating within 48 to 72 hours. Eat them soon thereafter, while they are still fresh and crisp. Whatever you don't eat, you can store in your refrigerator, where they will typically retain their freshness for up to a week. (If sprouts start to turn brown, as they often are when bought in a store, they are over-ripe and should not be eaten.) You can eat sprouts by themselves, or liberally sprinkle them atop salads, or add them to soups.

The following chart provides further instructions so that you can get started and make sprouts a part of your daily diet.

SPROUTING DIRECTIONS

TYPE OF SPROUT	SOAK TIME	RINSE/DRAIN TIMES	DAYS TILL EATING
Alfalfa	6 to 8 hrs	2X/day	3 days
Chickpeas	16 hrs	2 3X/day	3 days
Lentils	8 to12 hrs	2X/day	2 to 3 days
Mung beans	8 to12 hrs	2X/day	2 to 3 days
Sesame seeds	8 hrs	2X/day	1 to 2 days
Sunflower seeds	6 to 8 hrs	2X/day	1 to 2 days

Though sprouts are now widely available in most health food stores and supermarkets across the country, we recommend that you learn how to make your own sprouted foods. It is easy to learn how to do so (*see* How To Make Your Own Sprouts on page 81). By growing your own sprouted foods, you can be assured of their freshness, and have a constant supply of nutrient rich, highly alkalizing foods ready, available to you in your own kitchen.

The foods in this section should comprise the majority of every meal and snack you consume throughout the day. Especially concentrate on generous amounts of green, leafy, and colored vegetables, and consider adding sprouts to your menu selections to further boost your return back to acid-alkaline balance. Also be sure to drink adequate amounts of purified water or mineral water with a pH greater than 7.0. The charts in the next section will make it easier for you to make your food choices easily and wisely.

ALKALIZING AND ACIDIFYING FOOD TABLE

The following table categorizes the foods groups discussed in this chapter according to the degree (strong or mild) of alkalinity or acidity they produce in the body. Your goal is to create a daily diet that will optimize your body's ability to create and maintain proper acid-alkaline balance. To do this, you will want to eat as many of the alkalizing foods as you desire throughout the day, while minimizing your intake of acidifying foods, initially making them no more than 20 percent of your total food intake.

Obviously, it makes good sense to eat a lot of foods classified as very alkalizing, especially if you are suffering from chronic acidosis. These foods will produce more powerful alkalizing effects than foods that are only mildly alkalizing. Conversely, you will want to eat sparingly of foods that are very acidifying, choosing your acidifying foods from those that are only mildly so.

TABLE 4.2. PH EFFECTS OF FOOD GROUPS

BEVERAGES

STRONGLY ALKALIZING	MILDLY ALKALIZING	MILDLY ACIDIFYING	STRONGLY ACIDIFYING
Ginger tea	Almond milk	Beer (dark)	Beer (pale)
Vegetable juice (homemade, fresh-squeezed)	Apple cider	Coffee	Chocolate milk
	Apple juice (unsweetened)	Kefir	Espresso
	Coconut milk	Milk	Hot chocolate
	Green tea	Mineral water (carbonated)	Liquor
	Herbal teas	Wine	Milkshakes
	Mineral water (non-carbonated)		Soda
	Orange juice		Whiskey
	Pure water (Spring or filtered)		

FATS AND OILS

None	Coconut oil	Butter	Hydrogenated fats
	Flaxseed oil	Safflower oil	
	Olive oil	Sesame oil	
		Sunflower oil	

FRUIT

Blackberries	Apples	Dates	None
Cantaloupe	Apricot	Figs	
Honeydew melon	Avocado	Plums	
Kiwi	Banana	Pomegranates	
Lime	Blueberries	Tomatoes	
Mango	Cherries		
Papaya	Grapefruit		
Pineapple	Grapes		
Raspberries	Lemon		
Strawberries	Oranges		
Tangerines	Peaches		
Watermelon	Pears		

BREADS*

STRONGLY ALKALIZING	MILDLY ALKALIZING	MILDLY ACIDIFYING	STRONGLY ACIDIFYING
None	None	Dark bread (pumpernickel, wheat) Whole-grain bread (yeast-free)	White bread Yeast bread

*Note: If you choose to eat bread, you can neutralize its acidifying effects by toasting it. This helps to facilitate its digestion, placing less stress on the body. Avoid white bread altogether, however, including commercial hamburger and hotdog buns, as it is extremely acidifying. As a rule, bread should be eaten sparingly, if at all.

VEGETABLES

Artichokes	Asparagus	None	None
Beets and beet greens	Cauliflower		
Broccoli	Endive		
Brussels sprouts	Garlic		
Carrots	Onions		
Chicory	Peppers		
Cucumber	Radishes		
Dandelion greens	Shallots		
Escarole	Turnips		
Green beans			
Green cabbage			
Lettuce (avoid iceberg)			
Potatoes			
Red cabbage			
Spinach			
Squash			
Sweet pepper			
Sweet potatoes			
Yams			
Zucchini			

DAIRY PRODUCTS*

STRONGLY ALKALIZING	MILDLY ALKALIZING	MILDLY ACIDIFYING	STRONGLY ACIDIFYING
None	Butter, Raw, fresh	Cheese, soft (Brie, Camembert)	Butter, heated
	Buttermilk, fresh	Cheese, Provolone	Cheese, sharp (cheddar, Parmesan)
	Egg yolk	Cheese, Swiss	
	Milk, raw whole	Eggs, whole	Yogurt, sweetened
	Whey, fresh	Kefir	
		Milk, pasteurized	
		Yogurt, plain, organic	

*Note: Many people suffer from sensitivities to dairy products because they are lactose intolerant (lactose is a milk sugar). We recommend that dairy products be used sparingly, if at all.

LEGUMES (BEANS)*

STRONGLY ALKALIZING	MILDLY ALKALIZING	MILDLY ACIDIFYING	STRONGLY ACIDIFYING
None	Lentils	Chick peas	Soybeans
	Snow peas	Green peas	
	String beans	Kidney beans	
		Navy beans	
		Peanuts	
		Pinto beans	
		White beans	

*Note: The acidifying effects of legumes can be transformed into highly alkalizing properties by sprouting. For more on sprouts and how to make them, *see* page 81.

NUTS AND SEEDS

STRONGLY ALKALIZING	MILDLY ALKALIZING	MILDLY ACIDIFYING	STRONGLY ACIDIFYING
Chestnuts	Almonds	Pecans	Hazelnuts
Pumpkin seeds	Brazil nuts	Pine nuts	Soy nuts
	Cashews	Pistachio nuts	Walnuts
	Flaxseed		
	Hemp seeds		
	Macadamia nuts		
	Sesame seeds		
	Sunflower seeds		

GRAINS

STRONGLY ALKALIZING	MILDLY ALKALIZING	MILDLY ACIDIFYING	STRONGLY ACIDIFYING
None	Quinoa	Amaranth	Couscous
	Wild rice	Barley	
		Brown and white rice	
		Buckwheat	
		Bulgur	
		Millet	
		Oats	
		Rye	
		Spelt	
		Wheat	

MEATS, POULTRY, AND FISH

STRONGLY ALKALIZING	MILDLY ALKALIZING	MILDLY ACIDIFYING	STRONGLY ACIDIFYING
None	None	Bass	Bacon
		Chicken	Beef
		Flounder	Carp
		Haddock	Cold cuts/ processed meats
		Lamb	Crayfish
		Oysters	Hamburger
		Perch	Hot dogs
		Salmon	Lobster
		Sardines	Mussels
		Sole	Pork
		Trout	Veal
		Tuna	

FOOD COMBINING TIPS

In order to further enhance the health benefits of the above dietary recommendations we would like to add a few comments about food combining. The principles of food combining are based on the fact that the foods you eat are digested according to each food group's specific nature. For example, when we eat foods that are primarily high in proteins, such as meat, fish, or poultry, your body will digest it in the stomach. To do so effectively, your body needs to create a temporarily highly acidic environment.

By contrast, foods that are primarily high in starchy carbohydrates, such as breads, potatoes, or yams, begin to be digested in the mouth as you chew them. This process is then completed in the small intestines. For it to occur properly, a mildly alkaline environment is required.

Based on the above, it makes sense to avoid combining protein-rich foods with starchy carbohydrate foods during mealtime. By eating such foods in combination, your body is forced to attempt two entirely opposite tasks—digesting the protein foods in a highly acidic environment, while simultaneously digesting the starchy carbohydrates in an environment that is mildly alkaline. As a result, both food groups, when eaten together, will usually end up partially undigested. This means that your body will not be able to obtain the full supply of nutrients the food groups contain. Moreover, the undigested remnants will start to buildup in your colon, where they will decompose and ferment, creating toxins and mucus.

What follows are basic guidelines for food-combining that will make your meal choices easier and healthier.

- Eat protein-rich foods (meats, fish, poultry, and dairy) separate from starchy carbohydrates (potatoes, yams, breads, and wheat and grain products). Don't combine them together. This eliminates not only a meal of steak and potatoes, but also all-too-common lunch staples such as chicken salad, roast beef, tuna fish, or turkey sandwiches.

- Non-starchy carbohydrate vegetables (green, leafy, and colored vegetables), on the other hand, can be combined with either protein-rich foods or starchy carbohydrates. Such vegetables will not interfere with the digestion of either proteins or starchy carbohydrates.

- Fruits are best eaten alone away from meals. (With the exception of avocados and tomatoes, both of which can be included with meals.)

- Avoid drinking water with your meals, especially those featuring protein-rich foods, so as not to dilute the digestive juices needed to breakdown solid foods. Water is best consumed 20 minutes before eating, or 60 minutes afterwards.

- To further aid your body's digestive process, make sure you chew your food thoroughly before swallowing.

CONCLUSION

As this chapter makes clear, the primary cause of over-acidity that plagues our nation today is directly related to the abundance of acidifying foods that make up the standard American diet. By simply changing your diet to one that emphasizes alkalizing foods and following the guidelines we've presented in this chapter, you can significantly reduce the toxic burden of acidosis in your body easily and safely. It may take time before you see the results you are looking for—greater energy and freedom from disease symptoms—but with a little patience and discipline, you will begin to turn your health around simply by making sure your total food intake each day is comprised of meals containing at least 60 percent alkalizing foods.

For faster results, we recommend that you increase that percentage to 80 percent and ensure that you are drinking adequate amounts of pure water throughout the day. The importance of water to your health is covered in the next chapter.

5

Water
The Overlooked Healer

One of the easiest and most powerful things you can do for your health is to be sure and drink adequate amounts of pure, filtered water each and every day. That fact shouldn't be surprising. After all, approximately 70 to 75 percent of your body is composed of water. (In the bodies of babies, water composition is closer to 80 percent.) Because this is so, water is the medium through which all of your body functions occur.

Despite this fact, most doctors and health practitioners rarely consider whether or not their patients are meeting their daily water requirements, which is one of the reasons that so many people today *aren't* drinking enough water each day. Making matters worse, the standard American diet that most people in our country follow these days further interferes with the numerous functions that water helps your body perform. The end result is that many people are today chronically dehydrated and they don't even know it.

THE "WATER DOCTOR"

Water's numerous health benefits were clearly established by the late Dr. Fereydoon Batmanghelidj, who was recognized as the world's foremost authority on the relationship between water and health, and dehydration and disease. Dr. Batmanghelidj was a member of a prominent family in Iran, where he worked as a physician after receiving his medical training at London University's St. Mary's Hospital Medical School. In 1979, he was thrown into jail soon after the attack of the US Embassy by supporters of the Ayatollah Khomeini.

One night while he was imprisoned, prison guards brought another prisoner to his cell. The man was in pain because of a severe peptic ulcer. With nothing but water at his disposal, Dr. Batmanghelidj had the man drink two glasses of water. In less than ten minutes, the man's pain disappeared. Dr. Batmanghelidj then instructed him to drink two glasses of water every three hours, which he did, remaining pain-free for the remaining four months that he was kept captive.

Surprised by this success, Dr. Batmanghelidj went on to treat over 3,000 other cases of peptic ulcer during the nearly three years that he was imprisoned, conducting extensive research as he did so. So intrigued was he by his findings that he actually chose to continue his research in prison for an additional four months after he was scheduled to be released. When he finally left prison his research had already been written about in the *Journal of Clinical Gastroenterology* and the *New York Times Science* section.

Dr. Batmanghelidj, who passed away in 2004, spent the rest of his life exclusively studying and documenting how powerful water can be as a healing tool. He maintained that the primary cause of many illnesses was chronic dehydration, and his findings are reported in his books *Your Body's Many Cries for Water* and *You're Not Sick, You're Thirsty!* As he explained in his writings, since water is the medium that regulates all body functions, when we fail to provide our bodies with all of the water it requires each day to remain properly hydrated, over time many of our bodily functions become compromised and eventually damage and disease take hold.

Based on his many years during which he dedicated himself solely to researching the importance of water to overall health, Dr. Batman, as he liked to be called, became convinced that nearly everyone in the United States suffers from chronic, low-grade dehydration. His research also demonstrated that such dehydration played a primary role in many of the chronic diseases that beset our nation today and, more importantly, in many cases simply restoring the body to a properly hydrated state was enough to reverse these health conditions or, at the very least, reduce their symptoms. Yet, despite publishing his research and findings in medical journals both in the US and around the world, his work continues to be ignored by the medical profession. As a result, few people today understand the powerful positive difference that water can make in their health.

THE MANY ROLES THAT WATER PLAYS IN YOUR BODY

Perhaps the best way to explain why water is so important to your health is to point out that it is a solvent, which simply means that it can dissolve solids. Because of this fact, water is essential for regulating all of your body's functions, including the actions of all of the various solids that it transports, as well as oxygen molecules. Without water, your body would be deprived of the oxygen it needs. That's because oxygen, as it enters your body, is dissolved in water and then transported to all of your body's cells, tissues, and organs. When you are dehydrated, this process is impeded, leaving you oxygen deprived.

Your body also uses water to break down the food you eat into smaller particles. This process, in turn, enables the vitamins, minerals, and other vital nutrients foods contain to be metabolized and assimilated, while at the same time enabling food's unnecessary byproducts, or waste, to be eliminated. Without water, food has no energy value for the body. Simply put, without water, your body would soon die. And without *enough* water, many of your body's functions become impaired and in some cases suppressed. This is something that many people today are experiencing because they are dehydrated and don't realize it. Instead, they and their doctors often mistake the symptoms of chronic dehydration for various illnesses that they then seek to treat medically. In many cases, however, rather than medical treatments, all that is necessary is for patients to resupply their bodies with the water they need.

Water, along with oxygen, is also one of your body's primary sources of energy. It literally generates electrical and magnetic energy inside each and every one of your body's trillions, upon trillions of cells. This is especially important for healthy brain function, since the brain depends on an adequate water supply to operate. In addition, water also acts as a bonding adhesive that enables your cells to maintain their proper structure. Without enough water, cell structure cannot be properly maintained, leading to a loss of structural integrity and, eventually, disease.

Water also helps to prevent your body's DNA from being damaged and aids in its ability to repair itself. DNA (deoxyribonucleic acid) contains your genetic code and is found within each of your body's cells, keeping them healthy and properly functioning. When DNA becomes damaged it can cause cells to behave abnormally. Abnormal DNA is a known cause of cancer, as well as various other disease conditions. This means that, by drinking enough water each day, you can literally improve your resistance to cancer.

We hope the above points make clear to you why drinking plenty of water throughout the day is one of the best things you can do for your health. Yet water's health benefits do not end there. Here is a list of other roles water plays in your body. Water is essential for:

- generating electrical and magnetic energy inside each and every cell in your body

- maintaining the integrity of cell structure

- enhancing cellular DNA repair and preventing damage to DNA

- enhancing immune function, especially in bone marrow, where immune cells are formed

- increasing the ability and efficiency of oxygen collection in the lungs by red blood cells

- maintaining proper elimination and preventing constipation

- stabilizing and maintaining the health of the discs of the spine
- maintaining the health of the heart and overall cardiovascular system
- enhancing overall brain function (85 percent of your brain is composed of water)
- maintaining proper metabolism and digestion
- maintaining proper kidney and urinary function
- maintaining proper liver function
- maintaining proper regulation of body temperature via perspiration
- maintaining proper joint lubrication and muscle function
- maintaining healthy respiratory function
- maintaining proper function of the lymphatic system and the elimination of waste products via urine
- maintaining healthy functioning of the immune system
- maintaining healthy skin
- maintaining proper delivery of oxygen into the cells and the elimination of cellular wastes
- maintaining proper function of the body's "heating" and "cooling" systems
- maintaining proper production of your body's hormones and neurotransmitters

And that's still not the end of the benefits that water provides. Based on his many years of exclusively studying the relationship between water and good health, Dr. Batmangheldij found that drinking adequate amounts of water each day also helps prevent:

- addictive urges related to alcohol, caffeine, and various drugs
- anxiety, depression, and stress

- arthritis
- asthma
- attention deficit disorders in both children and adults
- back, joint, and muscle pain
- blood clots
- constipation and diarrhea
- edema
- fatigue
- gastrointestinal problems
- glaucoma
- heart disease
- high blood pressure
- hot flashes
- impotence and loss of libido
- infectious disease (due to boosting immune function)
- insomnia and other sleep problems
- kidney stones
- memory problems
- morning sickness during pregnancy
- PMS
- respiratory and sinus problems
- stroke
- urinary tract infection

Drinking adequate amounts of water each day is also one of the most potent ways that you can prevent and reverse one of our nation's most serious health scourges—obesity. Here's why.

HOW BEING CHRONICALLY DEHYDRATED CAN MAKE AND KEEP YOU FAT

Because of how essential adequate water intake is to its health, the human body sends out thirst signals as soon as its supply of water starts to run low. All of us are familiar with acute thirst signals that occur as the throat and tongue become dry and parched. For most of us, experiencing such symptoms is the only time that we may think to have a glass of water. But Dr. Batmanghelidj's research conclusively showed that relying on such acute thirst signals before drinking water is a big mistake. That's because such signals only arise after dehydration has already set in for many hours. And during all of that time, deprived of the water it needs, your body starts to experience a variety of significant, if initially unnoticeable, problems.

A Lack of Energy

One of the most common of these initial problems is a drop in energy. In fact, Dr. Batmanghelidj's research shows that most people who are habitually tired are simply dehydrated. Once their bodies are properly hydrated again, they very quickly regain their energy.

Similarly, many people who are overweight or obese are also chronically dehydrated. As most people who are overweight or obese can attest, they also tend to be tired most of the time. In fact, for many such people, a lack of energy often precedes unhealthy weight gain. Then, as more and more weight is put on, their energy levels plummet even lower, setting up a vicious cycle.

Based on Dr. Batmanghelidj's research, this fact is not surprising. As he and most other health experts have long known, an initial lack of energy in the body due to lack of water is quickly recognized by what Dr. Batmanghelidj termed the brain's "central control system." Because of how essential both water and proper energy levels are to the brain, once it senses a reduction of energy, it immediately sends out signals to the rest of the body to call upon its energy stores (primarily from calories stored in fat cells).

But, ironically, according to Dr. Batmanghelidj, these signals for more energy are where trouble lies. For, as he discovered, the body's "sensations of both thirst and hunger also stem from low ready-to-access energy levels."

As a result, as the brain sends out its signals for more energy, it also and at the same time sends out signals that create sensations of thirst and hunger, since water and food supply the body's energy needs. However, due to our modern lifestyle and dietary habits—both of which contribute to chronic dehydration—most people do not recognize the sensation of thirst for what it is, and therefore assume that the brain is only signaling for more food. That's because both thirst and hunger sensations are felt in the same areas of the body (the mouth and stomach area) and are both caused by the same thing—the release of histamine by the body. Thus many of us wind up eating when we should be supplying our bodies with more water instead. When we do, over time, we put on unwanted weight and the vicious cycle continues: We become more tired and then eat more than we need to as our brains and bodies cry out for more energy.

Why Drinking More Water Can Reverse This Deadly Process

To explain why drinking more water helps people lose weight, Dr. Batmanghelidj often pointed to the animal kingdom. Animals do not confuse the thirst and hunger signals from their brains. Instead they instinctively realize what both signals mean, and also give precedence to water over food. For these reason, animals in the wild always start their day by making an early morning visit to a water source. Only later, after they have consumed the water they require, do they turn their attention to eating.

By contrast, most people start their day by doing the reverse—eating first and only later getting something to drink. And usually it isn't water, but a cup of coffee in order to perk them up. By then, their bodies are already in for another day of chronic dehydration, which is only made worse by both the foods they eat and the coffee, which, for all its energy-giving properties, is also highly dehydrating. Then, as their day progresses and they find themselves getting tired, they again reach for food before water, perpetuating their health problems.

This unhealthy cycle could be easily reversed if people started their day by drinking two eight-ounce glasses of water 30 minutes before breakfast. People who need to lose weight should drink another two glasses of water 30 minutes before lunch and dinner, and another two glasses of water two hours after each meal.

This may sound like a lot of water, and for most people it certainly is, but the results speak for themselves. By following this simple recommendation, Dr. Batmanghelidj found that overweight and obese people soon found that they were able to better distinguish their thirst and hunger signals. Therefore, instead of eating more than they should, they were able to consistently eat less without trying because they felt full on less food, and they soon experienced more energy. Most importantly, they were also able to safely and consistently lose weight and keep it off without dieting or strenuous exercise. And, best of all, unlike the vast majority of people who find themselves regaining all the weight they lost after dieting, those who followed Dr. Batmanghelidj's advice were able to maintain their weight loss as long as they continued to drink enough water each day.

Since Dr. Batmanghelidj first published his scientific findings other researchers have confirmed what he taught. For example, researchers at the Franz-Volhard Clinical Research Center in Berlin Germany found that when men and women drank approximately 17 ounces of water, their metabolic rates (the rate at which calories are burned) increased by 30 percent within ten minutes after their water consumption. They also found that drinking more water improved the ability of men to burn fat, while increasing the ability of women to more efficiently metabolize carbohydrates

Based on their study, the researchers estimated that over the course of a year, people who increase their water consumption by 1.5 liters a day (approximately 51 ounces) would burn an extra 17,400 calories, and lose approximately five pounds.

So there you have it—one of the easiest and most effective weight loss solutions ever discovered. If you need to lose weight, drink more water!

HOW AND WHY WE BECOME CHRONICALLY DEHYDRATED

As we stated at the beginning of this chapter, many people today are chronically dehydrated and don't know it. Chances are, you could be one of them.

To get an idea of what happens to the cells and tissues of your body when dehydration sets in, consider a fruit set out on a countertop. If it is not eaten, before long it will begin to dry out, shriveling up both inside and out as it loses its water supply. Something similar happens to the cells and tissues in your body when chronic dehydration sets in. If not resupplied with water, the cells and tissues in the affected areas of your body will literally start to wrinkle, losing their structural integrity and their ability to function properly.

Factors Leading To Dehydration

It's no mystery why so many people are chronically dehydrated these days. After all, your body loses water each and every day simply through its daily activities. Adults lose an average of just slightly over three to four quarts of water every day due to activities such as breathing (exhalation), perspiration, urination, and elimination of bodily wastes. Breathing alone accounts for approximately one to two quarts of water loss each day.

Various factors can increase this water loss, as well. For example, people who are physically active or who exercise regularly experience more water loss than people who are sedentary. Water loss also tends to be higher among people who live at higher elevations. Fever and diarrhea can also increase the amount of water your body eliminates, as can perspiration due to high temperatures.

Based on what you've read in this chapter so far, it should be clear to you now that this lost water needs to be replaced each day if your body is to remain healthy. And the only way to do so is to drink more water and, to a lesser extent, eat more water-rich foods (certain fruits and vegetables).

Are You Dehydrated?

Prior to being educated about the important roles water plays in supporting good health, most people assume they simply need to pay attention to whether or not they feel thirsty to know if they need to drink more water. That's not the case. As previously stated, many people today often mistake their bodies' thirst signals as signs of hunger. This means they wait until their mouths become dry before thinking about drinking something. However, as Dr. Batmangheldij's research repeatedly showed, a dry mouth is actually the last outward sign that your body is dehydrated. That's because feelings of thirst don't develop until long after your body's water supply has fallen well below the level needed for optimal healthy functioning.

Rather than waiting until you feel thirsty, one of the easiest and most accurate ways to know if you need to drink more water is to monitor your urine.

- If your body has all the water it needs, your urine should be clear and colorless, and resembling unsweetened lemonade.

- If you are slightly to moderately dehydrated, your urine will generally be yellow.

- If you are severely, or chronically, dehydrated, your urine will generally appear orange or dark-colored.

■ **NOTE:** Urine can change color due to the use of vitamins and other nutritional supplements, often appearing bright yellow when such supplements are used.

Other telltale signs of dehydration are feelings of fatigue, dry skin, and joint and/or muscle aches and pains for no apparent reason, although all of these symptoms can also be signs of other health conditions.

WATER AND ACID-ALKALINE BALANCE

Water also plays a vital role in helping the body maintain its proper pH levels, especially with regard to the blood. In addition, water is essential for helping to eliminate acid wastes before they build up in your body's cells and tissues to cause health problems. It's more than likely that you've already experienced the benefits water can have in improving symptoms of acidity. For example, have you ever suffered from an "acid" stomach characterized by a burning sensation in your gastrointestinal tract? If you have, you probably reached for a glass of water and experienced relief of your symptoms after you drank it.

The Importance of Water—Being Hydrated

Unfortunately, most people fail to adequately keep their bodies hydrated. As a result, not only does the low-grade state of dehydration that ensues set the stage for the various health problems mentioned in this section, it also interferes with your body's ability to maintain proper acid-alkaline balance. Under normal conditions your body's blood supply contains an ample amount of water, which circulates over every one of your body's cell. Some of the water in blood enters into the cells, washing out acidity from them so that the cells' internal state remains a healthy alkaline environment. This is important for the health of your cells, and thus the overall health of your body.

Like blood itself, the interior of the cells requires a slightly alkaline pH of approximately 7.35 to 7.45 in order for cells to stay healthy. Only when the pH of the interior of the cells is at that level can the enzymes within the cells properly function. In addition, acid-alkaline balance within the cells is vitally important for the DNA within the cell nucleus, since this DNA is also alkaline and very susceptible to the damaging effects of acid buildup.

Only by keeping your body in a healthy, hydrated state can you ensure that your body's cells, along with the DNA and enzymes within them, stay healthy. Otherwise, acidity will begin to take hold within the cells, damaging their integrity and compromising the functioning of cellular enzymes and DNA.

The amount of urine you produce each day, as well as its color, is a good indication of whether or not you are drinking enough water and maintaining proper acid-alkaline balance within your cells and therefore your body. As Dr. Batmanghelidj wrote, "The more urine that is produced, the more easily the body keeps its interior alkaline. That is why clear urine is an indicator of an efficient acid-clearing mechanism, and dark yellow or orange urine is an ominous sign of impending acid burn in the interior of the body."

Water Quality Is Also Important

Sadly, in today's world, much of our water supply no longer has the neutral or slightly alkaline pH as that of water found in pristine areas of nature. Such healthy water has a naturally high content of alkalizing minerals, and also a high level of hydrogen ions, both of which play important roles in regulating acid-alkaline balance.

This fact was first discovered when scientists began studying the people of Hunza, a tiny region located in northwest Pakistan, in the Himalayan mountains. The Hunza people are famous for their excellent health and longevity, and commonly live to be 100 years old or more, free of bone loss, cancer, heart disease, and other chronic degenerative diseases that are the norm, rather than the exception, for elderly—and even middle-aged—populations here in the West. When scientists first began to research the Hunza people in the early twentieth century, one of the Hunza kings, when asked to explain the secret to his people's good health and longevity, replied, "It is the water." His claim was confirmed by the research conducted by Dr. Henri Coanda, a Romanian scientist famed for his work in the fields of both aeronautics and fluid dynamics. Coanda spent six decades studying the glacier-fed drinking water of the Hunzas, seeking to identify its health-giving features. He found that the surface tension of the water was low, making it highly absorbable. In addition, the water had a clustered crystalline structure that is similar to that of the fluids of the human body. And it was rich in both health-promoting minerals and a high concentration of active hydrogen known as hydroxyl ions, which increase the pH value of water. (When water carries more hydrogen ions than hydroxyl ions it is acidic. Conversely, a higher supply of hydroxyl ions compared to hydrogen ions makes water alkaline.)

Subsequent research by other scientists who have studied long-lived, healthy populations around the world have found that the water supply in those regions also have comparable properties as the Hunza water. Water from these regions is now recognized as the healthiest water in the world and for this reason it is sometimes referred to as "living water" because of its health-promoting qualities.

By contrast, much of the rest of the world's water supply can be consider to be "dead water," because it lacks such mineral content, has a low pH, and a higher supply of hydrogen ions than hydroxyl ions. One of the main reasons for this is because of how water is processed and delivered to municipalities, including the addition of harmful and acidifying elements such as fluoride, chloride, and other additives. This is why most tap water in the US not only does not have a neutral pH of 7.0, but actually a pH below that level, making it acidic.

Given that fact, it clearly makes no sense to drink water that adds to your body's acidic load as a means to flush out acids from your cells and tissues. In addition, many sources of tap water in the United States may also contain harmful microorganisms, including bacteria, fungi, and viruses. It is for these reasons that we recommend you drink only pure, filtered water or spring water known to be free of such impurities. (You can locate sources of spring water in your area by visiting www.findaspring.com, which maintains an updated list of spring water sources across North America.) You can also test the pH of your drinking water using the pH strips we discussed in Chapter 3.

To increase the alkalinity of your drinking water, you can use mineral drops, which are available at most health food stores, or add the juice of a fresh-squeezed lemon or lime. Or you can consider purchasing a home water ionizer unit. Such devices use a process of electrolysis to produce both alkaline and acidic water (acidic water can be used for skin care and is used in hospitals to treat skin wounds and infections; it is not intended for drinking). These types of devices have been shown to produce alkaline water similar to that consumed by the Hunzas. They were first developed in Japan in the late 1950s and were introduced to the United States in 1985. In Japan, Korea, and other Asian countries, these units are considered to be medical devices and are used in hospitals, as well as by tens of millions of Asians in their homes.

Because of the cost for such units (as well as the cost of their replacement filters), however, we don't regard them as being essential. What matters is drinking adequate amounts of water that is pH neutral or slightly alkaline each day, something you can easily accomplish using a water filter or by drinking spring or mineral water.

HOW MUCH WATER SHOULD YOU DRINK?

Based on his findings, Dr. Batmanghelidj advised that all of us should drink at least one-half ounce of water for every pound of our body weight. In addition, he also suggested that people consume a quarter teaspoon of salt per every 32 ounces of water drank per day, to help the body maintain an adequate supply of minerals. (Sea or Celtic salt is best, as these types of salt contain a much wider range of minerals than common table salt does.) The addition of salt increases water absorbability by the cells, thus enhancing water's ability to flush out acidic cellular waste.

As a general rule of thumb, Dr. Batmanghelidj recommended starting each day with two glasses of water and to drink water 20 minutes before eating food, although water with meals is permissible whenever one feels thirsty. Overall, we agree with these recommendations. Yet we also recognize that every person is unique and therefore has unique needs, including for the amount of water his or her body requires. For this reason, we recommend that you pay attention to your body and how it feels, and also monitor your urine. By doing so, you will soon begin to know for yourself how much water you should drink each day.

Here are some other guidelines we recommend you follow to keep your body properly hydrated.

- Drink pure, filtered water and avoid water in plastic bottles, as plastic contains unhealthy chemicals that can leech into water.

- Avoid drinking soda. In addition to being unhealthy for you, soda is also highly dehydrating. That same goes for commercial, non-herbal teas.

- Limit your consumption of coffee and alcohol, as both beverages are also dehydrating.

- Start your mornings by drinking a large glass of water before breakfast.

- Get in the habit of drinking a glass of water 20 to 30 minutes before each meal and another glass 30 to 45 minutes after eating. Doing so supports digestion and also reduces hunger pangs, leading to healthier eating habits.

- Take regular water-drinking breaks throughout the day, especially after each time that you urinate.

- Unless you are prone to waking up during the night to urinate, drink a glass of water before you go to bed.

CONCLUSION

Now that you've read this chapter, you know why water is so important to your health. We hope you act on this information by doing all you can to keep your body properly hydrated. If you do, we can promise you that will start to notice a positive difference in how you feel. These improvements will last so long as you keep drinking enough water each day. In the following chapter we look at the role certain nutritional supplements can play to further enhance acid-alkaline balance.

6

Helpful Nutrients

The dietary guidelines outlined in the previous chapter should serve as your primary means of restoring and maintaining optimal acid-alkaline balance in your body. But for most people, we also recommend the use of nutritional supplements to aid in this process. In this chapter, we will share with you the most important nutrients you can use to further enhance your overall health and aid in the recovery from over-acidity. First, though, let's discuss why we believe nutritional supplementation is so important.

Even if you eat fresh, organically grown food for all of your meals—something that is not necessarily easy to do for many people—such foods, although certainly richer in nutrients than non-commercial foods, are most likely still incapable of meeting all of your nutritional needs. There are two primary reasons why this is so. The first reason has to do with the constant stresses of daily life to which we are all exposed. Every day we are bombarded by stressors in the forms of difficult relationships (both at home and at work), noise and air pollution, and invading pathogens such as bacteria, fungi, and viruses. Some of us do a much better job of managing stress caused by such factors, but the one stressor to which we are all susceptible is chemical stress.

ROAD BLOCKS TO MEETING OUR NUTRITIONAL NEEDS

According to Drs. Robert Ivker and Robert Anderson, "Chemical stress may come from polluted air and water, food pesticides, insecticides, heavy metals, and even radioactive wastes. More than ever before, foreign chemicals can be found in our foods and environment. Many of these are commercially synthesized, but quite a few are naturally occurring as well." Your continued exposure to chemical stressors places a constant burden on your body as it works to maintain homeostasis. Because of this burden, the nutrients available from the foods you eat, as well as those that your body has stored up, can quickly become depleted. This is especially true of one of the most alkalizing minerals—magnesium. For this reason alone, daily supplementation with nutrients is a good idea.

But the challenge of achieving and maintaining your body's nutritional needs does not end there. Adding to the problem is the fact that today's soil in which food crops are grown contains significantly reduced levels of vital trace minerals. Because of the commercial farming methods used by today's agricultural industry, much of the trace minerals that had been abundant in our topsoil prior to the mid-twentieth century have been greatly depleted. To compensate for the poor condition of the soil, current farming methods rely on using substantial quantities of synthetic chemical pesticides, herbicides, and fertilizers to help crops grow. These commercial farming methods have been ongoing since the mid-twentieth century and have resulted in significant declines in the mineral content of food cropland, as well as declines in the overall nutrient content of the foods grown under such conditions.

Compounding the problem is the fact that much of our modern day food supply, after it is harvested, takes weeks and even months before it reaches us. Comparatively few of us eat locally grown food these days. Instead, the food that we consume, even if grown organically, is shipped from other parts of the country, frozen, stored, and warehoused along the way. This further reduces the nutrient content of food.

The final reason that we recommend supplementation, of

course, has to do with the burden of over-acidity that so many of us currently face. As we have discussed previously, in order to cope with over-acidity, your body draws from its stored mineral supplies, using those minerals to buffer and neutralize the effects of toxic acid buildup. The end result is not only over-acidity, but nutritional deficiencies as well.

With all of these factors working against us, you can understand why we feel that nutritional supplementation is so important. It just makes good sense to augment your diet with various nutritional supplements. Now let's take a look at the nutrients and other supplements we recommend you include as part of your daily health regimen.

ESSENTIAL NUTRIENTS FOR MAINTAINING PROPER pH BALANCE

To aid you in your journey to optimal health, we recommend daily supplementation of the following select group of vitamins, minerals, essential fatty acids, and digestive enzymes. When purchasing supplements, we also recommend that you choose brands comprised of food-grade concentrates (supplements containing nutrients derived from natural foods), as they are more useable in the body than the far more common synthetic brands.

A number of manufacturers provide food-grade multivitamin/multimineral formulas that contain adequate amounts of the vitamins and minerals as provided in this chapter. Read labels for more information, check to see if the supplement is food-grade, the dosage amount for each nutrient the supplement contains, and whether or not unnecessary fillers, dyes, and other non-essential ingredients are used (they shouldn't be). Once you are satisfied with the supplement's quality, follow the directions they contain for best results.

Essential Vitamins

Vitamins are required for the proper regulation of all of your body's many biological and metabolic functions. For the most

How to Read a Supplement Label

Before purchasing and using a nutritional supplement, it is important that you understand the quality of the product you are considering. In order to be better informed, we recommend that you always read the product label first. Here are some guidelines for doing so.

• Nutritional supplements (also known as "dietary supplements") include vitamins, minerals, herbs, essential fatty acids (EFAs), and other nutrients derived or synthesized from food sources. Such supplements, according to the Dietary Supplement Health and Education Act (DSHEA) of 1994, are not considered drugs and therefore are not required to be reviewed by the Food and Drug Administration (FDA) before entering the marketplace. However, the FDA does regulate what claims supplement manufacturers can make about their products, and this information is usually contained on the product label.

• Typically, product labels consist of a statement of identity, a structure-function claim, the form of product and net contents, directions for use, a supplement facts panel, a listing of other ingredients, and the name and address of the manufacturer. In the statement of identity you should find the brand name of the product and wording that clearly identifies the product as a "dietary supplement." This will be followed by the structure-function claim, which explains the health benefits of the nutrients the product contains, along with a required disclaimer saying, "This statement has not been evaluated by the Food and Drug Administration. This product is not intended to diagnose, treat, cure, or prevent any disease."

• Structure-function claims cannot say that a product or nutrient treats a disease, so be wary of any products for which such claims are made. But structure-function claims can state the role or function of the nutrient or nutrients in the body. For example, a multivitamin/multimineral formula with a structure-function claim stating "Helps support immune function" is perfectly acceptable. The federally required disclaimer means exactly what it says—that the FDA has not evaluated the claim, and no diagnostic, treatment, prevention, or curative claims can be made about the product in question. This is simply a formality in accordance with the DSHEA legislation.

- The form of product and net contents informs you about the form the product is in and the amount of its contents. Products can come in a variety of forms, such as capsule, tablets, liquid, or powder. If capsule or tablet forms are used, the label should tell you the amount of the product the capsules or tablets contain. If the product is in liquid or powder form, the total weight (usually ounces) will be listed.

- The directions for use on the label tell you how the product is intended to be taken. For example, the label may say, "Take one capsule daily." Pay attention to these directions and do not exceed the serving size of the product that is recommended.

- The supplement facts panel is something you should pay particular attention to. There, you will find the listed serving size (such as, one tablet or one capsule) of the product, as well as the active ingredients it contains, along with the amount of each ingredient per serving and the total percentage of the recommended daily intake (RDI) the product supplies for each nutrient. If an asterisk follows any of the ingredients, this means that no daily value has been established for that particular nutrient.

- The other ingredients listed supplies a complete listing of all the ingredients used in the formulation and manufacture of the product. Such ingredients will be listed in descending order, based on how much of each ingredient was used, with the most prevalent ingredient listed first, and the least prevalent ingredient listed last. Common ingredients in this listing include gelatin, water, binders, fillings, and coatings. Ideally, you should look for products that do not contain the last three.

- Finally, the label should supply you with the name and address of the product's manufacturer or distributor, including the zip code and, ideally, a telephone number or website address through which you can contact the company. If the product you are considering does not include all of the above information, we advise that you avoid purchasing it. And definitely be suspicious of any product that comes with a label claiming it can cure or treat a specific disease condition.

part, however, vitamins cannot be manufactured by the body, and therefore must be obtained daily through diet and supplementation. The most important vitamins with regard to proper acid-alkaline balance are vitamins A (as well as its precursor, beta-carotene), B6, B12, C, D, and folic acid.

Vitamin A and beta-carotene. Vitamin A is required for proper metabolism of calcium, a mineral with highly alkalizing properties. Vitamin A is also necessary to ensure good health of the eyes, skin, and teeth, and plays a key role in bone growth, cell differentiation, and tissue repair. It is also a potent antioxidant and important for proper immune function and protection against infectious disease.

Both stress and disease can diminish vitamin A stores, as can alcohol consumption, which we have already seen also has a significant acidifying effect on the body. Signs of vitamin A deficiency include night blindness, impaired bone and teeth formation, impaired immunity, and inflammation of the eyes.

One of the best ways to supplement with vitamin A is in the form of beta-carotene, which your body can convert to vitamin A in the liver. Beta-carotene is abundant in many colored and green, leafy vegetables, all of which are alkalizing, but since studies have found that nearly one-third of the American public consumes less than 65 percent of the recommended daily allowance (RDA) for vitamin A.

Dosage: We suggest supplementing with between 5,000 to 8,000 IU of either vitamin A or beta-carotene each day.

Vitamin B6. Vitamin B6, also known as *pyridoxine,* is involved in a wide variety of your body's internal processes, including immunity, energy-production, hemoglobin production, and the synthesis of proteins from amino acid. With regard to acid-alkaline balance, vitamin B6 plays two important roles. First, it helps regulate your body's sodium-potassium balance. Second, it aids in the delivery of magnesium inside of your cells. Both of these factors are essential for optimal energy production at the cellular level. An imbalance in sodium-potassium levels and/or a lack of cellular magnesium can have wide-ranging negative health effects and contribute to acidosis. Vitamin B6 also is required for production of hydrochloric acid (HCl), which helps your body digest and metabolize protein foods and also aids in the absorption of calcium. (For more information about HCl *see* page 240.)

Being water-soluble, meaning it cannot be stored by your body, supplies of vitamin B6, along with all other water-soluble vitamins (all B vitamins and vitamin C), can quickly be diminished. Signs of vitamin B6 deficiency include anemia, fatigue, headache, insomnia, muscle cramps and spasms, and nerve malfunctions. Though vitamin B6 is found in a variety of foods, such as bananas, cabbage, cauliflower, eggs, fish, poultry, organ meats, and whole grains, it can easily be destroyed due to commercial food processing and storage.

Dosage: Supplement with 2 to 5 mg each day, ideally as part of an overall, food-grade, vitamin B formula. For best results, take with meals.

Vitamin B12. The most important role vitamin B12 plays with regard to acid-alkaline balance is in proper bone growth and metabolism. Healthy bones are a sign that your body's pH levels are in balance, whereas bone loss is a sure indication of over-acidity. Vitamin B12 is essential for the cells that build bones to carry out their functions. Most importantly, vitamin B12 is also crucial for the development of the body's red blood cells.

Vegetarians are often deficient in vitamin B12 since it not found in significant amounts in fruits and vegetables. Signs of vitamin B12 deficiency include pernicious anemia, dizziness, fatigue, gastrointestinal disorders, low blood pressure, memory problems, moodiness, numbness, and vision problems. The best food sources of vitamin B12 are meats, fish, and dairy products, but since you will be limiting your consumption of such foods in order to achieve proper pH balance, it is a good idea that you daily supplement with vitamin B12.

Dosage: The current RDA for vitamin B12 is 3 mcg (lowered from 3 mcg in 1989), but many health experts deem this amount too low to meet your body's need for it. You should take at least 3 mcg of vitamin B12 per day.

Vitamin C. Vitamin C, also known as ascorbic acid, is one of the most important nutrients that your body requires because of the many and varied functions it plays a key role in. Besides being a potent antioxidant, it is essential for proper immune function and contributes to the health of bones, blood vessels, capillary walls, cartilage, joint linings, ligaments, skin, teeth, and vertebrae. It also is needed for proper wound healing, plays an important role in your body's detoxification processes, and enhances calcium absorption.

For all of its important functions, vitamin C is one of the least stable vitamins and can neither be manufactured nor stored by your body. Therefore, it is crucial that you receive adequate vitamin C intake each and every day. The best food sources of vitamin C include cherries, citrus fruits, dark green and leafy vegetables, green and red peppers, papaya, parsley, potato skins, and strawberries. It is not contained in any dairy, fish, poultry, or meat products.

Signs of vitamin C deficiency are numerous. They include anemia, bleeding gums, increased tendency toward bruising, lowered resistance to infections, mouth ulcers, and slow wound healing.

Dosage: Currently, the RDA for vitamin C is 60 mg, but most holistic health practitioners regard that amount as being extremely low. Take 3,000 mg of vitamin C per day, divided into three doses of 1,000 mg each spread throughout the day.

Vitamin D. Vitamin has recently been determined to act in the body more like a hormone than like a vitamin. It occurs in ten forms (D1-D10), but the two most important form as a nutritional supplement is D3. Regular exposure to sunlight can help your body manufacture its own vitamin D supply. For most people, however, because their lifestyle affords them little time outdoors, they are often unknowingly deficient in vitamin D.

Vitamin D's most important role in helping to maintain acid-alkaline balance has to do with the way it aids in the absorption of calcium and in regulating the metabolism of both calcium and phosphorous. In doing so, it also enhances the health of your bones and teeth. Other functions that vitamin D aids includes regulating the nervous system, maintaining the health of the cardiovascular system, and maintaining normal blood clot function.

Signs of vitamin D deficiency include bone softening (osteomalacia), hearing loss, nearsightedness, osteoporosis, psoriasis, and tetany (a form of muscle spasm). Good food sources of vitamin D include butter, cod liver oil, egg yolk, liver, milk, and oily fish, such as herring, mackerel, sardines, and salmon. As mentioned, vitamin D can also be synthesized by your body following exposure to direct sunlight. Ideally, try to expose at least one-third of your body (arms, face, and hands) to sunlight for 20 to 30 minutes each day.

Dosage: As a supplement, take between 800 to 1,000 IU of vitamin D3 a day.

Folic acid. Folic acid is also known as folate and vitamin B9. In addition to aiding in the production of red blood cells and helping to regulate proper cell division, folic acid is also needed by your body to properly metabolize sugars and for the production of neurotransmitters (chemical substances necessary for communication between nerve cells). It also plays a key role in helping to detoxify homocysteine from the bones. Homocysteine is a waste product created when the amino acid methionine is metabolized, and when it is not properly eliminated it can lead to both artherosclerosis and osteoporosis.

The best food sources for folic acid are dark green vegetables, eggs, nuts, and organ meats. Research shows that folic acid deficiency is quite common, due to such factors as poor diet, drug and alcohol abuse, and stress. Signs of deficiency include anemia, diarrhea, fatigue, gastrointestinal disorders, headache, irritability, palpitations, and general weakness.

Dosage: Folic acid deficiency is common, therefore we recommend supplementing with 400 mcg each day, preferably as part of an overall food-grade, vitamin B formula.

Essential Minerals

Minerals are often overlooked when it comes to nutritional supplementation. They should not be, especially since mineral deficiencies are widespread within the soil our food crops are grown in, making for mineral-deficient fruits, vegetables, and grains. This is a trend that began in the early 1900's, and which has become far worse over the last few decades due to the widespread use of chemical fertilizers and other harmful chemicals used in the production of our nation's food crops.

Minerals play many vital roles in the health of your body, working in conjunction with vitamins, enzymes, hormones, and other nutrient co-factors to regulate numerous biological functions. These include proper blood formation, energy production, regulating bodily fluids, metabolic processes, nerve transmission, and maintaining the health of bones and teeth. Minerals are also key regulators of proper acid-alkaline balance. The most important minerals in this regard are boron, calcium, copper, magnesium, phosphorous, potassium, silica, and zinc.

Boron. Boron is important to acid-alkaline balance because it helps your body metabolize and make use of various other nutrients, such as calcium, vitamin D, and magnesium, all of which also play roles in maintaining healthy pH levels. Boron also contributes to the overall health of the bones, which is where your body stores much of the minerals it uses to buffer and neutralize acid buildup. Recent research suggests that boron helps regulate your body's endocrine system, which is responsible for how your body produces and makes use of hormones.

Potential signs of boron deficiency include diminished levels of the hormones estrogen and testosterone, both of which are essential for healthy bones and osteoporosis. Among older women, boron deficiency can also contribute to problems related to post-menopause.

Dosage: Currently, there is no established RDA for boron intake. Fortunately, adequate levels of boron can be obtained solely from your diet, by eating plentiful amounts of fruits, nuts, and vegetables. We recommend this approach over supplementing with boron because taking more than 3 mg of boron as a supplement can interfere with your body's ability to make use of its calcium supplies, whereas boron obtained from foods, even in much higher levels, does not cause this problem.

Calcium. Among all minerals, calcium is the most abundant mineral in your body. Nearly all of it–99 percent—is stored in bone tissue, where it is used to ensure the health of both bones and teeth. Your body uses the remaining one percent of its calcium supply to help regulate blood clotting and blood pressure levels, cardiovascular function, cell division, and muscle and nerve function. Calcium is also required for healthy skin. It is one of the primary acid-buffering minerals called upon by your body whenever excess acids pose a problem.

It is important to supply your body with adequate amounts of calcium each and every day, ideally through your diet. Unfortunately, the standard American diet is severely lacking in calcium. This is not surprising given the chronic state of acidosis such a diet creates.

The most familiar signs of calcium deficiency are bone and skeletal problems. Of these, the most common are fracture and osteoporosis. Other symptoms include anxiety, brittle nails, depression, insomnia, muscle cramps, diminished nerve function, and problems related to teeth.

According to Dr. Susan Brown, a leading medical anthropologist, Americans derive 80 percent of their calcium supply from dairy foods, whereas in other parts of the world, the primary sources of dietary calcium are vegetables (especially broccoli, collard greens, and dark green leafy vegetables), and certain types of fish, such as sardines and salmon. Almonds and Brazil nuts, both of which are also alkalizing foods, are other good food sources of calcium. These nondairy sources of calcium are far more absorbable, and therefore meet a greater percentage of your body's daily calcium needs. Given that fact, as well as how acidifying a diet high in dairy products can be, we strongly suggest that you make vegetables your primary food source of calcium, along with the nuts and fish.

Since the 1980s, calcium supplements have been recommended to women by physicians and other health experts as a means of preventing osteoporosis. Recently, however, the advisability of calcium supplementation has been called into question by research indicating calcium supplements can increase the risk of calcification of the arteries and, therefore, heart attack and stroke. Interestingly, calcium obtained from foods does not pose this same health risk.

Dosage: We strongly advise you to meet your body's calcium requirements through the calcium-rich foods listed in this section.

Copper. Copper is an essential trace mineral that is found in all body tissues, and is especially concentrated in the liver and brain. Among its various functions, copper helps in the manufacture of hemoglobin, and with the synthesis of oxygen in red blood cells. It also plays a role in helping to regulate insulin levels and helps prevent unhealthy weight gain. Recently, scientists discovered that copper is necessary for healthy bones, as well.

Despite its importance to health, copper is one of the most noticeably lacking minerals among most Americans. This is especially true of people who follow the standard American diet, which contains only 50 percent of the RDA for copper. Symptoms of copper deficiency include anemia, dermatitis, edema, fatigue, impaired respiration, and tissue and blood vessel damage.

Dosage: Like boron and calcium, copper is best obtained through food sources, since the RDA for copper is only 1.5 to 3 mg. The best food sources of copper include dark leafy green vegetables, eggs, lamb, legumes, pecans, oysters, poultry, and walnuts. In order to help create proper pH balance, we recommend making dark leafy green vegetables a staple food source for meeting your daily copper needs.

Magnesium. Approximately 65 percent of your body's magnesium stores are found in your bones and teeth, followed by high concentrations in your muscles. Magnesium is also contained in the blood and other body fluids, as well as inside your cells. It plays many roles in your body, including participating in hundreds of enzymatic reactions and acting as a musculoskeletal relaxant. Magnesium is also important for the health of your heart, and for preventing heart attacks because of its ability to relax coronary arteries and, just as importantly, for its role in cellular energy production in the form of ATP (Adensosine Triphosphate). (Your heart has the highest need of ATP of any organs in your body.)

Magnesium also aids in proper cell division, cell maintenance and repair, hormone regulation, proper nerve transmission, protein metabolism, and thyroid function. Magnesium also helps the body assimilate and use calcium and vitamin D, and is necessary for healthy bones and teeth.

Though often undiagnosed, magnesium deficiency is very common among Americans due to a variety of factors, such as poor diet, copper-deficient crops, overcooking of foods, and overconsumption of alcohol. In fact, most experts in the role magnesium plays in overall health consider nearly the entire population of the US to be deficient in magnesium.

Symptoms of magnesium deficiency include depression, fatigue, gastrointestinal disorders, hypertension, irregular heartbeat, memory problems, mood swings, impaired motor skills, muscle spasms, nausea, and osteoporosis. The best food sources of magnesium are dark green vegetables, which are also highly alkalizing and rich in chlorophyll. Other good food sources include apricots, avocado, brown rice, legumes, nuts, seaweed, and seeds.

As we stated earlier in this book, magnesium in the body is particularly susceptible to depletion because of stress. Because of how easily magnesium can be depleted in the body and because of how prevalent stress is in our society, we recommend a multipronged approach for meeting your daily magnesium needs. First, be sure to eat an abundant supply of magnesium-rich foods each day (doing so will also enhance acid-alkaline balance). Then consider using both magnesium supplements and topical magnesium oil, especially during times of elevated stress. Finally, take a relaxing Epsom salt bath once or twice a week. To enhance your body's ability to use oral magnesium supplements, take them along with vitamin B6.

Another form of magnesium supplementation, known as magnesium oil in the form of magnesium chloride, has gained popularity. Instead of being taken orally, magnesium oil is absorbed through the skin after it is topically applied. According to Dr. C. Norman Shealy, topical magnesium oil is one of the best ways to ensure that your body obtains all of the magnesium it requires because of how quickly this form gets absorbed by the cells.

Dosage: Daily supplementation of magnesium is vitally important for your overall health, as well as for maintaining proper acid-alkaline balance. The late Dr. Mildred Seelig, one of the world's preeminent researchers of magnesium's many health-giving properties, recommended that adults multiply their body weight by five, and then take that amount of magnesium in milligrams (mg) each day. For example, a man weighing 200 pounds would require 1,000 mg of magnesium, whereas a women weighing 120 pounds would require 600 mg of magnesium per day. Since magnesium can have a laxative effect when taken in high doses, it is best to divide your magnesium supplemental intake per take into two to three doses, taken with meals. For general use, the best absorbed oral forms of magnesium are magnesium glycinate and magnesium malate.

You can also obtain magnesium from Epsom salt baths. Simply add one to two cups of Epsom salt to a bath of hot water (as hot as you can comfortably tolerate) and soak your body for 30 to 40 minutes.

Dr. Shealy's research has shown that topical magnesium oil, applied once or twice per day (one to two ounces at a time) can result in optimal cellular levels of magnesium in as little as 30 days, compared to six months for oral magnesium supplements. The only inconvenience of using magnesium oil is the oily residue (hence its name) that it leaves on the skin once it is applied. For this reason, we recommend that you apply magnesium oil 20 minutes before you shower, as 20 minutes is the minimum time required for enough of the magnesium to be internally absorbed. Then you can shower off the remaining residue.

MSM. MSM (*methyl sulfonyl methane*) is a sulfur compound that naturally occurs in our bodies. When adequately available, it helps your body build healthy cells and enhances the health and growth of your hair, muscles, nails, and skin. It also plays an important role in the manufacture of collagen, the primary component of your body's cartilage and connective tissue.

In recent years, MSM has gained a reputation as a natural means of alleviating pain related to arthritis, based on studies which showed that arthritis patients who supplemented with MSM experienced significant improvement in their symptoms. Additional research indicates that MSM can increase hair and nail growth and help repair damaged skin. It also enhances the ability of body fluids to more easily pass through tissues, thus improving the delivery of oxygen and nutrients to the cells, and the elimination of cellular waste products.

Though MSM is available in fresh fruits and vegetables, meats, milk, and seafood, most people are deficient in sulfur because of how the body continuously uses and excretes it. This deficiency is made worse by the fact that all too often people do not eat enough MSM-rich foods and, even when they do, levels of the compound are often still lacking due commercial food harvesting, processing, and packaging methods. In addition, MSM levels in the body naturally decline with age. As they do so, the risks of fatigue, organ and tissue malfunction, and susceptibility to disease all increase. Supplementing with MSM is an effective and inexpensive way to ensure your body abundantly meets its daily sulfur requirements.

MSM is an extremely safe and nontoxic substance, very similar to water in this regard, as it is almost impossible to consume too much of it. Your body will use what it needs and eliminate what it does not.

Dosage: We recommend that you supplement with between 2,000 to 5,000 mg of MSM daily, depending on your specific nutritional needs. For best results, take it with meals, along with vitamin C.

Phosphorous. Phosphorous is the second most abundant mineral in your body, exceeded only by calcium. Like calcium, it is primarily concentrated in the bones and teeth, although it is found in every body cell. It is involved in nearly all of your body's biochemical reactions. Among its many functions, phosphorous helps form DNA and RNA; aids in cell communication, growth, and repair; and plays a vital role in energy production. It also is essential for good bone and teeth health, heart function, muscle and nerve function, and the metabolism of B vitamins, calcium, fat, glucose, and starch. It is one of the most important minerals that your body draws upon to buffer and neutralize acid buildup, and therefore is essential for proper pH balance.

Although phosphorous deficiency is considered rare, phosphorous stores can easily be depleted due to the use of antacids and lack of vitamin D. Symptoms of phosphorous deficiency include anxiety, arthritis, impaired bone growth, irritability, and general weakness. Health problems can also occur when phosphorous levels exceed those of calcium and, conversely, when levels of phosphorous are too low compared to calcium levels.

The best food sources of phosphorous are protein-rich foods, such as cheese, eggs, fish, milk, meats, and poultry. Nuts, seeds, and whole grains are other good sources.

Dosage: Given the rarity of phosphorous deficiencies, we recommend that you obtain phosphorous primarily from your diet, but caution against consuming too much protein-rich foods due to their acidifying effects. By following the 80 to 20 alkaline to acid rule discussed in Chapter 5 (*see* Page 89), you can avoid this problem.

Potassium. Potassium is an essential body salt. Approximately 98 percent of your body's potassium stores are found within the cell membranes. Potassium helps conduct bioelectrical current throughout the body, maintains cellular integrity and fluid balance, and helps regulate nerve function. It also aids in energy production and heart function. Inside the cells, potassium also regulates water and acid-alkaline balance, making it crucial for proper pH levels.

Potassium deficiency is quite common among most Americans—especially among our aging population. It is also common among people who suffer from chronic illness. One of the main causes of potassium deficiencies, besides poor diet, is our nation's over-reliance on diuretics and laxatives, both of which strip potassium from the body. Eating canned and processed foods can also deplete potassium supplies because of their high sodium (salt) content. Symptoms of potassium deficiency include arrhythmia, depression, fatigue, hypertension, hyperglycemia, mood swings, and impaired nerve function.

The best food sources of potassium are fresh fruits and vegetables. Bananas, in particular, are rich in potassium. Other good food sources include nuts, seeds, whole grains, and fish, such as salmon and sardines.

Dosage: Though there is no established RDA for potassium, most people require between 2,000 to 5,000 mg per day. A variety of potassium supplements are available, in the forms of both tablets and liquid. Either form is well-absorbed.

Silica (Silicon). Silica, also known as silicon, is the most abundant mineral on earth. In your body, it is primarily concentrated in the arteries, collagen, connective tissue, eyes, hair, ligaments, nails, skin, teeth, and tendons. Silica is important to pH balance because it helps make other minerals, particularly calcium more bioavailable. This, in turn, helps maintain strong and flexible bones. It also ensures that adequate calcium stores are available when your body needs to draw upon them to buffer and neutralize acid buildup.

Signs of silica deficiency include atherosclerosis, fatigue, lowered resistance to infectious disease, and diminished strength of bones and teeth. Because of how important silica is to the health and integrity of connective tissue, its lack can result in unhealthy skin, especially in terms of elasticity. Joint problems can also be related to silica deficiency.

Silica is widely available in the fibers of most fresh fruits and vegetables, grains, nuts, and seeds. However, since fibers are stripped during commercial food processing, people who eat a diet high in processed foods will usually be deficient in silica.

Dosage: The RDA for silica has not been established, but research indicates that at least 20 to 30 mg of silica per day is required to maintain good health.

Zinc. Zinc is one of the most important minerals that your body needs to ensure its health. In addition to being a potent antioxidant, zinc is necessary for your body to properly perform over two hundred enzymatic reactions. It also is important for detoxification, bone repair, maintaining healthy cellular membranes and tissues, ensuring proper immune function, and regulating insulin production. Zinc also helps your body absorb and utilize vitamins A and D and calcium. In men, zinc is essential for the health of the prostate gland.

Zinc deficiencies among Americans are quite common. Vegetarians are particularly susceptible to zinc deficiency. Lack of zinc can result in dermatitis, fatigue, hair loss, impaired immune function, loss of libido, and osteoporosis. It can also increased risk of prostate problems, including enlargement, infection, and prostate cancer. The RDA for zinc is 15 mg for adults, although many health researchers believe this level is far too low. We recommend 30 to 45 mg per day, especially for men over 40 years of age.

The best food sources of zinc include beef, egg yolk, herring, nuts, and shellfish. Whole grain bread also contains zinc. However, given the large number of people who suffer from wheat allergies or sensitivities, it is not an optimum food source in my opinion, especially as breads are also highly acidifying.

Dosage: When supplementing with zinc, it is best to take it in the form of picolinate for optimum absorption. Since zinc can interfere with your body's ability to absorb and utilize copper, it is best to take these supplements apart from each other.

Essential Fatty Acids

Though excess fat consumption can lead to a variety of health problems, your body requires certain types of fat each day in order to be healthy. These fats, which are not produced by your body, and therefore must be obtained through diet and supplementation, are known as "essential fatty acids" (EFAs). They are called "essential" because of the many important roles they play in the body. EFAs help your body produce energy, regulate hormone and nerve function, and maintain healthy brain function. They also aid in overall musculoskeletal function and calcium metabolism, and help to reduce inflammation in the body. EFAs make up a part of cell membranes and are particularly concentrated in the adrenal glands, brain cells, the eyes, nerve cells, and the sex glands. There are two primary forms of essential fatty acids—omega-3 fatty acids and omega-6 fatty acids.

Omega-3 fatty acids. These occur in three forms, alpha-linoleic acid (ALA), docosahexanoic acid (DHA), and eicosapentaenoic acid (EPA). DHA and EPA are found in various cold-water fish, such as mackerel, salmon, and sardines, while ALA, which acts as a precursor to both DHA and EPA, is contained in healthy oils, such as fish oil and oils derived from flaxseed, hemp, pumpkin, and walnut. Flaxseeds, pumpkins, and walnuts by themselves are also good sources of omega-3 fatty acids. Since your body has to convert ALA into DHA and EPA, we recommend that people who suffer from illness or weakness obtain omega-3 fatty acids from fish, as this spares the body from having to expend energy in the conversion process.

Dosage: An easy way to meet your omega-3 EFA requirements is to take a capsule containing both EPA (300 mg) and DHA (200 mg) once a day.

Omega-6 fatty acids. The primary forms of omega-6 fatty acids are gamma-linolenic acid (GLA) and linoleic acid. Both forms of are found in black currant, borage seed, primrose, safflower, and sunflower oils, as well as fish oils. Almonds and pumpkin seeds are other good sources.

EFAs in the form of omega-3 and omega-6 fatty acids provide a number of health benefits. One of the primary benefits has to do with cardiovascular health. EFAs help to reduce and eliminate the presence of saturated fats and other toxins in the arteries, thus helping to prevent atherosclerosis and minimizing the risk of unhealthy blood clots. In addition, they reduce cholesterol, low-density lipoprotein (LDL), and triglyceride levels, all of which are directly associated with heart attack, hypertension, and stroke, as well as atherosclerosis.

Other benefits of EFAs include improved metabolism of fats, more efficient energy production, and better regulation of insulin. Other conditions that have shown improvement when optimal EFA levels are obtained from the diet or through supplementation include alcoholism, arthritis, diabetes, eczema, kidney and liver problems, multiple sclerosis, premenstrual syndrome (PMS), and skin problems. More recent research also suggests that EFAs may play a role in inhibiting the growth and spread of cancerous tumors.

Ideally, it is best to obtain all your EFAs from the foods and oils mentioned above. However, due to the importance of EFAs to health, supplementation may also be advisable. EFA supplements are commonly available in capsule form. If you choose this option, make sure the capsules are fresh. To be certain, break one capsule open and smell it. If you notice a foul odor, do not consume it.

Dosage: To ensure that you are receiving an adequate supply of omega-6 EFAs, take 1,000 mg of evening primrose oil.

Digestive Enzymes

Digestive enzymes are derived from plants and play a similar role in the body as the enzymes contained in fruits and vegetables. (Other food groups do not contain enzymes.) Such enzymes are essential for proper digestion. They become active in the stomach, where they aid in predigestion of food as it is consumed, enabling your body to more efficiently assimilate the nutrients the foods contain. Increasingly, physicians and health practitioners are advising their clients and patients to use digestive enzyme supplements for better health.

Enzyme Deficiencies and Their Causes

In an ideal environment, you would derive all of the enzymes your body requires for proper digestion from the foods you eat. All fruits and vegetables contain an abundant supply of enzymes, but in today's world, even eating large quantities of such foods is not enough to ensure that you are obtaining all the enzymes your body needs. One reason for this is that enzymes are heat sensitive and are destroyed when foods containing them are cooked in temperatures above 118 degrees F. Microwaving food also destroys enzymes. For this reason, it is best to eat fruits and vegetables raw or lightly steamed.

Numerous other factors can also cause enzyme deficiencies. Chief among them are many of the commercial farming and food production methods used to harvest and deliver so much of our food supply. Such methods include the use of chemicals and pesticides; gene-splicing, genetic engineering, and hybridization; irradiation; and pasteurization, all of which deplete enzyme supplies in fruit and vegetable crops. Canning food destroys enzymes, as well.

According to noted enzyme expert Lita Lee, Ph.D, author of *The Enzyme Cure,* other factors that can cause enzyme deficiencies include high intake of unsaturated and hydrogenated fats, drinking fluoridated water (which is also absorbed by the skin during bathing and showering), and exposure to radiation and electromagnetic fields, such as those emitted by computers and television screens. People who have mercury amalgam dental fillings and/or root canals can also suffer from enzyme deficiencies, according to Dr. Lee, due to the harmful health effects such dental procedures can cause. Heavy metal toxicity, a condition that is far more widespread than most people realize, depletes enzyme activity, as well. For all of these reasons, supplementing with digestive enzymes is a good idea.

We also recommend that you consider supplementing with digestive enzymes with all of your meals. Doing so will not only help you better digest the foods you eat and better assimilate the nutrients they contain, it will also aid in your body's energy production. The enzymes we recommend are all plant-based, meaning they are derived from raw fruits and vegetables. The primary plant-based enzymes are amylase, cellulase, disaccharidase, lipase, and protease. Your body is capable of manufacturing enzymes similar to each of these enzymes except cellulase, which can only be obtained through food or through supplementation.

Amylase. Amylase digests carbohydrates. Amylase deficiencies can result in incomplete digestion of carbohydrates. In addition to lack of amylase from food sources, sugar consumption can also result in amylase deficiency.

Like other enzymes, amylase performs more than one function in your body. In addition to carbohydrate digestion, amylase helps ease muscle soreness following physical exertion, and can also help relieve stiff joints and conditions, such as writer's cramp. It also helps to prevent and eliminate the buildup of dead white blood cells known as leukocytes, which can turn into pus and cause abscesses in the body. Amylase is also helpful in preventing and managing allergic reactions, canker sores, fungal infections, gallbladder and liver problems, herpes, hives, lung conditions such as asthma and bronchitis, and skin rash. Foods such as whole grains, raw fruits and vegetables, and raw nuts are good sources of amylase.

Cellulase. Cellulase is essential for the proper digestion of fiber, which it helps the body convert into usable glucose for energy. Since no enzyme similar to cellulase is manufactured by your body, it is important that you eat cellulase-rich foods. The best food sources are raw fruits and vegetables, as well as whole grains. Besides helping to digest fiber, cellulase also digests yeast and fungi, making it useful as an aid in preventing and relieving candidiasis (systemic yeast infection), as well as bowel and vaginal yeast infections. It also helps digests certain neurotoxins related to facial pain and paralysis, and is very effective in neutralizing intestinal bloating and flatulence. Cellulase is also effective in stopping acute food allergies. Foods such as avocado, oat sprouts and peas are good sources.

Disaccharidase. Disaccharidase plays a vital role in the digestion of sugars known as disaccharides. The three primary forms of disaccharides are lactose (milk sugar), maltose (grain sugar), and sucrose (cane sugar). Disaccharidase breaks these sugars down into glucose and fructose, which your body can make use of more efficiently. Eating refined sugar, which is a staple of the standard American diet, is the primary cause of disaccharidase deficiency.

Disaccharidase can be helpful in relieving the physical and mental/emotional symptoms caused by sugar intolerance. Physical symptoms of sugar intolerance include dizziness, gastrointestinal conditions, and respiratory problems, particularly asthma. Mental/emotional symptoms include anxiety and depression, attention deficit disorder (ADD), bipolar disorders, hyperactivity, mood swings, and panic attacks. Disaccharidase can also help mitigate symptoms associated with lactose intolerance, such as constipation and diarrhea, and help reverse the spread of candidiasis.

Lipase. Lipase is the enzyme your body requires in order to digest fats, primarily tryclgycerides. In addition, lipase enzymes play an integral role in maintaining cell wall permeability. This permeability allows nutrients to easily pass into your body's cells, and for cellular wastes to pass out from the cells to be eliminated.

Lipase deficiency is fairly common. It occurs primarily in people who have an intolerance of fats and in people who are intolerant to complex carbohydrates. Because of their intolerances, both groups can eventually become deficient in lipase. Such people have a higher risk of developing atherosclerosis and other cardiovascular problems, chronic fatigue, diabetes, gallbladder problems, high cholesterol, hypertension, and varicose veins. They are also more prone towards excessive weight gain and obesity, and more apt to suffer from deficiencies of fat-soluble vitamins, such as vitamins A, D, and E. Good food sources include coconuts, flaxseeds, soybeans, spinach, and wheat germ.

Protease. Protease, when taken with meals, digests proteins into amino acids, which are essential for the growth, maintenance, and repair of your body's tissues. It is also required for energy production and optimal mental function, as well as many other physiological processes. Protease, when not taken with meals, also digests the protein coating of bacteria, viruses, and other microorganisms, making them better able to be identified and eliminated by the immune system. It is their protein coating that makes such pathogens elusive to your body's immune factors. Protease also helps to protect against blood clots, and can help eliminate them should they form.

When protease is lacking in the diet, incompletely digested proteins can result in low blood sugar (hypoglycemia), and in an overly alkaline pH in the bloodstream. The first condition is due to the fact that approximately half of the protein you consume, when it is properly digested, is converted into useable sugar. Properly digested protein also helps to ensure proper acid levels in the blood. When protein digestion is incomplete, the blood takes on excessive alkaline reserves, forcing the kidneys to work overtime to excrete them into the urine. This buildup of excess alkaline reserves, according to Dr. Lee, can often result in a state of anxiety. Other conditions can then benefit from protease supplementation, including appendicitis, arthritis, bone spurs, bacterial and viral infections, immune problems, kidney problems, and osteoporosis. A good food source of protease is papaya, guava, ginger root, spinach, wheat, and kidney beans.

GUIDELINES FOR USING NUTRITIONAL SUPPLEMENTS

Unless otherwise indicated, take nutritional supplements with meals. This will aid in their absorption, making it easier for your body to derive the benefits such supplements can provide. Fat-soluble nutrients, such as vitamins A, beta carotene, and essential fatty acids (EFAs), should be taken with the meal of the day that has the highest fat content, to enhance their effectiveness.

If you are taking high dosages of nutrient supplements, be

sure to do so with your physician's full awareness and approval. In such cases, do not take the dosages all at once, but divide them up throughout the day. Doing so will make it easier for your body to make use of them.

The following are other guidelines we recommend when taking nutritional supplements.

- Take mineral supplements away from high-fiber meals, as fiber can interfere with your body's ability to absorb minerals.

- When supplementing with individual B vitamins, also supplement with a complete vitamin B-complex supplement, as B vitamins work most effectively in concert with each other.

- Avoid supplements that contain artificial sweeteners, binders, coatings, fillers, fructose, or preservatives.

If you are also using prescribed medications, be sure to inform your physician about your nutritional supplement use, as certain nutrients and herbs can interfere with certain pharmaceutical drugs and possibly cause adverse side-effects.

CONCLUSION

While no amount of nutritional supplementation can replace the role that a healthy diet can play in your health, there is no question that the supplements discussed above are important. This is especially true whenever you find yourself struggling with over-acidity and the health conditions associated with them. By eating and supplementing wisely, and by following the general dietary recommendations we covered in Chapter 5, you can make steady and significant progress in your journey to vibrant health.

Now let's look at another factor that can play a significant role in helping your body to maintain a healthy pH-balanced state—your breath. You may think you are breathing properly and therefore don't need to learn more about breath, but more than likely you are not. To find out why, read on.

7

Restoring Acid-Alkaline Balance With Your Breath

Here's a statement that will probably surprise you: *If you are like most people, you aren't breathing correctly.* You might be asking yourself how we could say such a thing. After all, isn't breathing something that everybody does automatically and unconsciously all the time?

Yes, and that's where the problem lies, because most people not only are not conscious of how they breathe, they also don't realize that they are breathing inefficiently. Are you one of them? To find out, take a moment and perform the following simple exercise.

- Sitting normally, place one hand over your chest and one hand over your belly. Now breathe the way you normally do, without changing anything, keeping your attention focused on your hands.

- As you inhaled, which hand moved? If you are like most people, the answer is the hand you placed over your chest. (If your answer is the hand you placed over your belly, congratulations! This means you are breathing more efficiently than the vast majority of people today.)

- If the hand over your chest is the one that moved, you are a "chest breather," meaning you habitually breathe in and out of

Meet Your Respiratory System

The simple act of breathing involves a complex, interwoven network of organs known as your respiratory system. It is comprised of your nose, sinuses, larynx and trachea (your throat), bronchi, and your lungs and has two primary purposes: supplying life-giving oxygen to each and every of the trillions of cells in your body, and expelling carbon dioxide and related waste byproducts. In the process, it also plays a significant role in helping to regulate and maintain your body's acid-alkaline balance.

To accomplish these tasks, during the course of the day (24 hours) you inhale approximately 22,000 pints of air each day. As you do so, your nose and sinuses (the sets of air-filled cavities around your nose and eyes) act as protective air filters, preventing airborne particles such as dust, soot, and smoke, as well as harmful microorganisms from moving deeper into your body. Your nose and sinuses also act as a biological humidifier and regulator of body temperature. As necessary, they moisten dry air, cool hot air, and warm cool air that would otherwise shock and potentially harm your lungs.

Your entire respiratory system also has a protective outer lining known as the respiratory epithelium. This single, continuous tissue stretches from the inside of your nostrils down to alveolar sacs in your lungs. Its outer tissue, known as the mucous membrane, or mucosa, continues the filtration process begun in your nose and sinuses, trapping any microorganisms or particulate matter that may escaped their protective mechanisms. This task is primarily performed by microscopic hair-like filaments known as cilia. It is due to a breakdown of mucosal function that colds, flu, and other respiratory conditions are able to take hold in the body.

There are two types of breathing, or respiration: external and internal. External respiration refers to the intake of oxygen and the exhalation of carbon dioxide. Internal respiration, also known as cellular respiration, refers to the process by which glucose and other molecules within the cells are supplied with oxygen to produce energy. It is during this process of energy production that carbon dioxide is produced as a by-product.

your chest. This is not the ideal way to breathe, since chest breathers tend to take short, shallow breaths, and as a result they do not take in as much oxygen with each inhalation or exhale as much carbon dioxide and other waste products compared to "belly breathers."

Another serious downside of chest breathing is lack of energy flowing through your body. Fortunately, this pattern is very easy to break with a little attention and effort.

THE RELATIONSHIP BETWEEN BREATHING, HEALTH, AND ACID-ALKALINE BALANCE

In addition to supplying oxygen, removing carbon dioxide and helping to maintain pH balance, breathing is involved in a variety of other life-supporting activities (*see* Meet Your Respiratory System on page 132). It helps to rejuvenate blood vessels and stimulates the heart via the oxygen it supplies, thereby protecting and maintaining healthy cardiovascular function. It also plays a role in optimizing brain and cognitive function.

All of the processes that occur as we breathe do so automatically, which is why most of us take our breathing for granted. That is until our respiratory system becomes compromised. And that is something that happens all too often in our society due to such factors as air pollution, smoking, and secondhand exposure to cigarette smoke. But other, less obvious internal factors can also impair respiratory function, such as impaired immunity, stress, poor diet, spinal misalignments, chronic muscle tension, the overuse of pharmaceutical drugs, and being overweight, which is a common cause of sleep apnea, a condition characterized by regular periods of breath cessation during the night.

Recent research has also found that a different type of apnea occurs during acts of typing and while reading emails and during Internet browsing. Since most of us today primarily type when we are writing emails, this condition is now referred to as "email apnea," a term first coined by Linda Stone, a former Apple executive who discovered that approximately 80 percent of the population, when engaged in writing tasks, tend to regularly pause their breathing or breathe shallowly as they do so, triggering a "fight or flight" response in the body's sympathetic nervous system.

Inefficient breathing habits compound all of these problems and impair the various functions that breathing plays in your health. And as we mentioned at the top of this chapter, it's highly likely that you currently have such habits to some degree. People who habitually take shallow breaths into the chest, along with pauses in their respiration, are unknowingly contributing to a host of potential health problems, starting with a lack of energy due to a lack of oxygen, first in the cells, and then in the heart, brain, and other organs. This, in turn, results in a buildup of acidic wastes within the body's cells, tissues, and bloodstream, disrupting proper acid-alkaline balance.

Far more than water or food, the oxygen you breathe is your most important supply of energy. In fact, without an adequate supply of oxygen from breathing, your body is unable to efficiently and fully metabolize food and water so that they provide their numerous health benefits, regardless of how healthy the quality of the food and water is that you consume. You can follow the healthiest diet in the world, but if you aren't supplying your cells with an abundant supply of oxygen your health will still remain less than optimal.

Poor breathing habits not only impair your body's ability to balance pH and perform all of its many other functions, it also increases the burden caused by accumulating acidic wastes that remain in your cells and tissues because of how improper breathing patterns prevent such wastes from being completely eliminated during exhalation. Most people, when they think of how wastes are eliminated from their bodies, erroneously assume that the primary methods of elimination occur in the bowels and bladder. In actuality, only about 30 percent of elimination of bodily wastes occurs this way. The other 70 percent, including carbon dioxide and related by-products, is eliminated through breathing.

Simply put then, *poor breathing habits result in poor elimination, which in turn results in an ongoing buildup and accumulation of wastes in your body.* Since such wastes are acidic in nature, this means that your body has to work harder to maintain its acid-alkaline balance. And, because breathing is a primary mechanism for maintaining this balance, poor breathing habits creates a vicious cycle whereby additional acidic wastes continue to accumulate inside your body at the same time that one of the main ways your body has for dealing with such wastes—breathing—is inefficiently doing its job. Just as excessive, rapid breathing (hyperventilation) causes alkalosis (over-alkalinity), shallow breathing (hypoventilation) causes acidosis.

Research has established that suboptimal breathing and the buildup of cellular waste that results from it is also related to one of our nation's most serious health problems—obesity. The reason for this is twofold. First, diminished breathing predisposes the body to increase fat production. Second, when toxins build up in the body beyond the body's capacity to eliminate them, the uneliminated wastes are shunted by the body away from its vital organs to be stored in fatty tissues, especially in the thighs, waist, and upper arms. This storage causes additional fat buildup in the body and eventual weight gain and its associated discomfort and lack of energy. This, in turn, makes it even more difficult for the body to perform as nature intended, due to the additional loss of energy, thus making it harder for proper pH balance to be maintained, as well as negatively impacting a wide variety of other biological functions.

Researchers at the National Institutes of Health (NIH) have also found that poor breathing habits, including pauses between breaths, significantly increases the risk for stress-related illnesses precisely because of the acidity that such breathing habits cause. Moreover, the researchers found that poor breathing places a burden on the kidneys by causing them to reabsorb sodium, and also causes imbalances in the body's levels of oxygen, carbon dioxide and nitric oxide (NO), a compound that helps to regulate inflammation in the body, and which plays an essential role in the immune system's ability to fight bacterial, viral, and parasitic infections, as well as tumors. Additionally, NO is a vasodilator, meaning that it expands the arteries, therefore improving blood flow, and in males it also plays a significant role in preventing erectile dysfunction. It also helps transmit messages between nerve cells and plays a beneficial role in brain functions associated with learning and memory. It also aids in healthy sleep, helps relieve pain, and is vital for healthy heart function.

Another major way in which poor breathing habits negatively impact our health has to do with a major nerve in your body called the vagus nerve. Extending from the head down through the neck into the chest and abdomen, the vagus nerve is actively involved in regulating the two branches of your body's autonomic nervous system—the sympathetic and parasympathetic nervous systems. The sympathetic nervous system is associated with the body's "fight or flight", or stress response, while the parasympathetic system is associated with the relaxation response, rest, and healthy digestion. It governs your sense of hunger and fullness, as well as the flow of saliva and digestive enzymes.

Research has shown that deep, relaxed breathing habits cause the vagus nerve to signal the parasympathetic system to become dominant, triggering non-stressful states of relaxation. Shallow, inefficient breathing, on the other hand, activates the sympathetic nervous system and the "fight or flight" response, which in turn causes the liver to spill glucose and cholesterol into the bloodstream, accelerates heart rate, and diverts energy away from other biological functions in anticipation of a biological perceived need to deal with dangers associated with the stress response. Chronic poor breathing habits, therefore, result in a chronic state of stress in the body. As we previously pointed out, chronic stress rapidly depletes stores of magnesium, a primary alkalizing mineral, thus further impairing your body's ability to maintain healthy pH levels.

BECOME A BETTER BREATHER

The primary reason why so many of us habitually breathe inefficiently is because we are unconscious of our breathing. Yet breathing is the only ongoing function our bodies perform over which we have conscious control. Simply by paying attention to our breathing empowers us to breathe more efficiently and fully. This is one of the reasons why so many meditation techniques are based on focused, conscious breathing, since conscious breathing helps to create states of "in the moment" awareness.

Like meditation itself, however, initially becoming conscious of your breathing patterns can seem difficult, especially given all of the other things we need to pay attention to as we go about each day. Fortunately, the benefits of conscious breathing do not require you to constantly focus on your breathe to be attained. Rather, research shows that they can be attained in as little as 20 to 30 minutes a day. Moreover, this short time frame can be divided into smaller 3 to 5 minutes "breathing breaks" during the day. What is important is to make sure that you *do* get into the habit of breathing deeply and fully for at least a few minutes each and every day. And, since you can do so regardless of whatever else you may be doing, focused breathing is something you can do anywhere and at any time.

In the remainder of this chapter, we are going to share with you some of the most effective and easy-to-perform breathing exercises you can choose from each day in order to counteract the health-ravaging effects of shallow breathing. We recommend that you experiment with all of them, and then choose the ones that you most enjoy and perform them on a daily basis.

Belly Breathing

The primary characteristic of shallow, inefficient breathing habits is inhalation that occurs in the chest. Typically, such breaths are short. If you performed the exercise that opened this chapter, you already know whether or not you are a "chest breather." If you are, the following exercise will help you quickly experience what it feels like to breathe through your belly (diaphragm). Diaphragmatic, or belly, breathing is how singers are trained in order to achieve maximum lung function.

Place your elbows on a table, desk or windowsill, leaning forward as you do so. Once in this position, take a deep breath in through your nostrils. (Always inhale and exhale through your nose and not your mouth, because it is your nostrils that warm and moisturize air before it reaches your lungs. Breathing in through your nose instead of your mouth also pulls air deeper into the lower parts of your lungs, allowing for a greater exchange of oxygen into the rest of your body.)

As you breathe while in this position you will discover that your inhalation naturally and automatically begins in your abdomen, with little to no movement occurring in your chest cavity. You will also notice that you are taking in more air with each inhalation than you normally do when you breathe in through your chest. Stay in this position and continue to breathe for a few minutes. As you do so, don't be surprised if you start to feel more relaxed and also more energized. Such experiences are a natural consequence of "belly breathing."

For some people who habitually breathe primarily through their chest, getting accustomed to breathing in through the belly may at first feel uncomfortable. If this is the case with you, just recognize it for what it is—a shift away from your normal comfort zone. Instead of giving up, continue to experiment with belly breathing on a daily basis. As you do so, you will soon find your discomfort fading away, to be replaced by increased feelings of calm and energy.

By making it a habit to breathe in through your belly whenever you focus on your breath, you will soon find that these positive feelings will become more and more a part of your daily life. More importantly, by choosing to take deep, relaxed breaths through your belly, you can quickly and effectively dissipate many of the effects caused by stress. Best of all, you can afford yourself of these benefits at any time, simply by breathing in through your belly wherever you are and whatever you are doing. Before long, you will find that your breathing has become deeper and fuller, with each breathe supplying you with greater amounts of oxygen. Eventually, you will also likely discover that your breathing is expanding your rib cage and relaxing any muscle tension in your upper torso that you may previously have been experiencing.

Belly breathing is the foundation of greater respiration. Not only is it a far more efficient way to breathe than breathing in through the chest is, it also goes a long way to maintaining the dominance of your body's parasympathetic nervous system, thereby benefiting all of your body systems that have energy diverted away from them when your body moves into "fight or flight" mode when the sympathetic nervous system is dominant. We encourage you to make belly breathing a habit, and to also take belly breathing breaks throughout the day, ideally for a few minutes each and every hour. During that time, simply focus on breathing in and out through your belly for two to five minutes at a time.

■ **NOTE:** As you begin to practice belly breathing, as well as the other breathing exercises in this chapter, be sure not to overdo it in order to avoid hyperventilation. Gradual progress is best, because too rapid a change in your breathing habits, especially hyperventilation, can lead to uncomfortable side effects.

In addition, our recommendation for belly breathing does not mean you should not breathe in and out through your chest. Rather, we want to emphasize that the most effective way for you to breathe is to start your inhalation deep within your abdomen. The more that you practice belly breathing, the more the musculature of your upper torso will relax. Over time, you will find yourself quite naturally beginning your inhalation in your belly and ending it high up in your chest without any need for straining. Once you do so, you will have achieved a much greater level of control over your breathing. The health and other benefits that you reap by doing so make the time and effort necessary to reach that point more than worthwhile.

A Breathwork Visualization

As we mentioned, focused breathing is a primary component of most meditation techniques. Visualization is another common element of many meditation techniques. The following exercise combines both elements. Performing it will not only further help you start to breathe more efficiently, it will also increase your energy levels and help to release tension in your body caused by stress.

Here's how to perform it:

1. Sit straight and comfortably, with your feet flat on the ground.

2. Close your eyes and focus on your breath. Gently begin to breathe deeply in and out from your belly.

3. Each time you exhale mentally tell yourself, "Relax." Do this for a few moments, until you feel a wave of relaxation starting to move through your body.

4. Now place your attention on your head, jaw, and face. As you continue breathing, visualize and direct the wave of relaxation throughout all of the muscles of your face and jaw, including those of the eyes, then over your scalp and along your head, down to the base of your neck, telling each part of your head, face, and jaw to relax as you exhale.

5. Repeat this process with each remaining part of your body, beginning with your shoulders, back, arms, and hands, then moving down to your chest, abdomen, pelvis, thighs and upper legs, calves, ankles, feet, and toes. Be sure each area of your body becomes more relaxed before you move your attention to the next area.

6. Once you have proceeded all the way to your toes, continue to sit with your eyes closed for a few more minutes, still breathing gently in and out of your belly, allowing your feelings of relaxation to deepen.

7. Just before you open your eyes, allow your breathing to become deeper and fuller, feeling a wave of energy passing through you. Once you feel vitalized, open your eyes and return to your daily activities.

We recommend that you initially spend five minutes performing this exercise. Over time, you may find yourself naturally extending the time you spend doing it to ten minutes or more. Good times for performing it are upon awaking in the morning, during your lunch break, or prior to going to bed. Try to perform it at least once a day, and even more during times that are particularly stressful for you.

Retained Breathing

This breathing exercise helps to improve metabolism and increase energy due to the way in which it enhances the exchange of oxygen from the lungs into the bloodstream. The greater exchange of oxygen helps cells to more efficiently receive more of the oxygen and nutrients carried by the blood and to more effectively eliminate carbon dioxide.

To perform this exercise:

1. Start by sitting in a chair in a relaxed manner, keeping your spine straight. Your eyes can remain open or closed.

2. Once you are seated and ready, take a deep breath in through your belly. At the end of your inhalation, hold your breath for a count of three. Then exhale fully. At the completion of your exhalation, again hold your breath for a count of three. Then inhale once more and repeat this entire process ten times. If at first you have difficulty doing this, you can reduce the count for both the inhalation and exhalation down to two, or even one, then work your way back up to three.

3. As soon as you are comfortable holding your breath for a count of three on both the inhalation and exhalation increase the hold to a count of five, then, when it is comfortable for you to do so, to a count of ten.

4. When you can comfortably hold your breath for a count of ten after each inhalation and exhalation, gradually increase how long you hold your breath after each inhalation (*only after each inhalation*) until you can do so for a count of 20 to 30 (*no more than 30*), while still holding your breath after each exhalation for a count of ten. This increased breath holding after each

inhalation is the primary reason why this exercise is so effective at enhancing oxygen exchange in the lungs.

For best results, go slow and pay attention to your body, only increasing how long you hold each breath when it feels comfortable to do so, and make sure each inhalation begins from your lower belly. Once you achieve the 30:10 breath-holding ratio between each inhalation and exhalation, you can perform this exercise for five minutes once or twice each day. Doing so over time will increase your lung capacity (something that tends to otherwise decrease as we age), boost your metabolism, and leave you feeling more energized, making it an excellent "pick-me-up" during times of fatigue.

■ **NOTE:** While holding your breath can increase acidosis, this exercise only does so very briefly, while at the same time helping you to increase your lung capacity and thus your overall oxygen intake. In short, the long-term benefits of this exercise far outweigh the fleeting shift towards acidosis that can occur while you retain your breath.

Alternate Nostril Breathing

This breathing technique was developed thousands of years ago and is an exercise that is well known to practitioners of yoga. It originated as a basic breathing technique within an aspect of yoga known as *pranayama*. *Prana* is a Sanskrit term for vital life force energy, just as *Qi* ("chee") is within the field of traditional Chinese medicine (TCM), which includes the practices of Tai chi and Qigong. The term *pranayama* means "regulation of *prana*" and involves the control of the breath in order to enhance the flow of energy throughout the body.

According to yogic tradition, alternative nostril breathing (known as *nadi shodhana*, a Sanskrit term meaning "purification of the channels," or *nadi*, which are similar to the meridian energy pathways of TCM) purifies the energy pathways through which *prana* flows throughout the body, balancing both the breath and vital energy.

Before beginning alternate nostril breathing, you might want to try another simple experiment. Place a small mirror beneath your nose and exhale. Now look at the condensation left on the mirror. Most likely, one circle will be larger than the other, meaning that more breath is passing in and out of the nostril in question. During the day, you will find that the nostril with the larger degree of air flow also alternates. Practicing alternate nostril breathing over time will minimize this discrepancy and improve how your central nervous system functions. The benefits of this cannot be overstated, since your nervous system affects every cell and body system in the body.

Alternate nostril breathing is performed as follows:

1. Sit up straight, with your spine, neck, and head aligned (*see* Breathing and Your Spine on page 144). When you are comfortable, begin to breathe in a relaxed manner through your belly. Do so slowly three times, keeping your inhalations and exhalations for the same duration.

2. After completing your third breath, inhale once again and then, before you exhale, close your right nostril with the thumb or index finger of your right hand, and exhale completely through your left nostril. As you complete this exhalation, release your right nostril and close your left nostril, then inhale through your right nostril.

3. Repeat this pattern of exhaling through your left nostril and inhaling through your right nostril for a total of three times, keeping the length of time of each exhalation and inhalation the same.

4. At the end of your fourth inhalation through your right nostril, exhale through the same nostril while keeping your left nostril closed. Then repeat the above process, only this time by inhaling through your left nostril and exhaling through your right nostril. Do this for three times as well.

5. When you finish, place your hands comfortably on your knees and exhale and inhale through both nostrils for three more times. This completes this exercise.

In the beginning you may find that you have to strain a bit more while inhaling through one of your nostrils. That simply indicates that at that moment you are taking in more air from the other nostril. With time, this discrepancy will also disappear.

It is recommended that you perform this exercise on a daily basis, both in the morning and before you go to bed, and more often during the day if you wish. Doing so will help to balance the flow of energy throughout your body. Some yoga teachers also claim that it will aid in synchronizing the left and right hemispheres of the brain, contributing to greater alertness and enhanced cognitive abilities.

Breathing and Your Spine

One of the most overlooked aspects of health is the health of your spine, even though musculoskeletal disorders such as back pain are among the most common health complaints. A healthy spine plays a far greater role in overall health than most people suspect. Not only does a properly aligned spine minimize the risk of musculoskeletal disorders, it also ensures optimal function of the nervous system, which regulates all of the body's other systems. It does so by using the network of nerves that branch out from your spinal cord to extend to every organ and gland in the body.

When your spine becomes misaligned—a condition known as "subluxation"–the nerve impulses transmitted by the brain become impaired. This results in diminished function on the part of the body systems to which the brain sends its messages. The primary structural cause of nerve interference is pressure placed on the nerves by misaligned vertebrae. (The spine consists of 24 vertebrae, from which the spinal nerves extend outward to the rest of the body.) Chronic muscle tension, muscle spasm, and constricted connective tissue within the musculature, can also contribute to this problem, by pulling and keeping the vertebrae out of alignment. Once the spine is restored to its

Twenty Connected Breaths

This technique was developed by Leonard Orr, the founder of a breathing process known as *rebirthing* or Conscious, Connected Breathing. Rebirthers maintain that learning to breathe with awareness without pausing between the inhale and the exhale can result in a variety of physical, psychological, and spiritual improvements while also improving the quality of our thoughts and releasing limiting and erroneous personal beliefs.

In this exercise, you may notice a tingling sensation in all or part of your body. For some, this can be uncomfortable, but the

proper alignment, nerve function improves, resulting in improvements in the rest of the body's systems, as well.

Misalignments in the spine, along with associated muscle tension, also significantly interfere with your ability to breathe fully in a deep, relaxed manner. Full respiration is very similar to a wave motion in which all parts of the respiratory system, as well as the musculoskeletal system that supports it expand and contract in a fluid, uninterrupted manner. Spinal misalignments impede this full range of motion, decreasing air intake and forcing the body to expend more energy and effort in order to breathe deeply.

Incorporating a regular program of stretching or other exercises designed to promote flexibility is an excellent way to help maintain proper spinal function. Such exercises also incorporate the breath, making them ideal forms of self-maintenance. If you suffer from spinal misalignments, there are a number of healthcare treatments that can help you address the problem. The most popular of these are chiropractic, bodywork and massage, and osteopathic manipulation. Other therapies, such as yoga, tai chi, Rolfing, the Alexander Technique, and Bowen Therapy, can also be most helpful. Becoming aware of and addressing spine and muscle tension can lead to dramatic long-term improvements in your overall health.

feelings will quickly become pleasurable if you allow yourself to simply keep breathing.

The exercise is performed as follows:

1. Once a day, preferably upon arising or before going to bed, take four short breaths with your mouth closed, remembering not to pause between the inhale and the exhale. Do not force the breath, especially on the exhale, which should simply release of its own accord. On the fifth breath, inhale and exhale deeply and fully. These five breaths together count as one cycle.

2. Repeat three more times for a total of four cycles and 20 connected breaths.

Breathing in this manner can sometimes bring up suppressed feelings and unpleasant thoughts or memories. If you find this to be the case, don't give up. As you continue to practice this exercise, such experiences will resolve and you may find, as they do so, that you gain meaningful insights into why they arose, usually ending with a sense of resolution of the issues in your life they are associated with. If you are interested in receiving deeper instruction in rebirthing breathwork you can find more information, as well as a directory of practitioners trained in this method, by visiting www.rebirthingbreathwork.com.

Laughter, Yawns, and Sighs

Not many people realize it, but laughter is actually one of the most effective ways of breathing because of its ability to short-circuit all of our standard defense mechanisms. Besides triggering a greater breath response, research has shown that laughter—especially bouts of unbridled laughter—also relieves physical tension and stress, leaving your muscles relaxed for up to 45 minutes afterward. Laughter also increases the activities of immune cells and infection-fighting antibodies, thus improving your resistance to disease, and releases a flood of endorphins, your body's natural feel-good chemicals. Research also shows that laughter helps to diminish pain, relax muscles, and improve the function of blood vessels while enhancing blood flow, thus helping to protect against heart attack, stroke, and other cardiovascular problems.

Laughing often throughout the day is a sure sign that you are increasingly becoming healthier on all levels on your being. So here's to the latest hilarious joke you hear. Be sure to spread it around!

Similarly, yawning and sighing can also increase your intake of breath and can be marvelous ways of relieving stress and rechanneling energy, as well. Whenever you feel the urge to do one or the other, heed the urge and do so. You may find the experience becomes even more pleasurable and invigorating if you exaggerate it.

CONCLUSION

In summary, breathing is the most important physiological act we can perform. Be aware of how you breathe, experiment with your breath, and notice how breathing deeply leaves you feeling more relaxed and happy. As all sacred scriptures teach, the Breath of Life is our divine birthright, so breathe in and out with all the gusto you can muster. The more that you do so, the more relaxed and energized you will begin to feel, and the greater control you will have over daily sources of stress. For more about stress and how to manage it, turn to the next chapter.

8

Coping With Stress

According to the Centers for Disease Control and Prevention (CDC), stress is the primary cause of 85 percent of all diseases. Research by health experts, such as Stanford biologist Dr. Bruce Lipton and other researchers in the field of mind/body medicine, also known as psychoneuroimmunology (PNI), indicates that the CDC's figure is too conservative, with their findings showing that stress is a major factor in over 95 percent of all cases of disease in the United States.

These numbers are backed up by even more startling statistics.

- An average of one million US workers miss work every day due to stress-related disorders, and up to 75 percent of all lost work time each year is directly due to stress.

- As much as 80 percent of all industrial accidents are due to stress.

- Ninety percent of all visits to primary care physicians in the US are directly due to stress-related complaints.

- According to a landmark 20-year study conducted by researchers at the University of London, unmanaged stress is a more serious risk factor for both heart disease and cancer than either cigarette smoking or frequent consumption of high cholesterol foods.

How Stressed Are You?

The following questionnaire can help you find out how well you are coping with stress. It is comprised of a list of symptoms and behaviors associated with chronic stress exposure.

Review this list and check off all symptoms that you may currently be experiencing.

___ Anger that persists

___ Anxiety/worry that persists

___ Back, neck or shoulder pain/stiffness/tension

___ Biting your nails

___ Change in your sense of taste

___ Cold hands or feet

___ Constipation

___ Diarrhea

___ Difficulty concentrating

___ Difficulty swallowing

___ Digestive problems

___ Dizziness

___ Excessive belching

___ Fatigue that is persistent

___ Frequent colds

___ Headaches

___ Heartburn that persists

___ Heart palpitations/racing heartbeat

___ Hemorrhoids

___ High blood pressure

___ Indecisiveness

___ Insomnia

___ Itchy or "burning" skin

___ Loss of appetite

___ Nausea

___ Nervous exhaustion

___ Persistent feelings of loneliness, sadness, and/or unworthiness

___ Oversleeping

___ Sexual problems

___ Shortness of breath

___ Stiff or painful muscles and/or joints

___ Trembling

___ Unexplained stuttering/ stammering

_____ **Total number of checks**

> Add up the number of items you checked on the list above. This will give you a better idea about how well, or poorly, you are coping with stress. (Obviously some of the items on this list can also be due to other causes, yet even then stress is very likely to be a co-factor.) If you checked off ten or more items, then we recommend you seek the help of a stress counselor or other health professional trained in stress management techniques.

However, despite the compelling scientific evidence linking stress to illness, little attention to managing stress is usually given by doctors when they consult with their patients. Although doctors may counsel their patients to try to relax more, rarely do they provide them with effective self-care tools for doing so. Instead, they may prescribe tranquilizing drugs, which can provide temporary relief, but do not address the underlying problem.

Fortunately, there is much that you can do on your own to better manage stress, starting by following the recommendations in this book. In this chapter, we want to add to what you have already learned by showing you why unmanaged stress can severely impact your health, and then provide you with the tools you need to take control over the sources of stress in your life.

HOW STRESS LEADS TO DISEASE

All of us are exposed to stress each and every day. Without stress, life as we know it would not be possible. This is because certain types of stress are essential for good health. For example, when you exercise your muscles, you are placing them under stress. In this example, such stress is a positive thing, because it causes your muscles to become stronger, leading to improved strength. Stress also plays a role in stretching and aerobic exercises, also leading to a healthy effect.

In short, your body is designed not only to cope with a certain amount of stress, but also to actually *depend* on some level of stress for its survival. As another example of this fact, consider what happens to astronauts who spend extended periods of time in states of reduced gravity and, in some cases, weightlessness. As they do so, they begin to lose muscle strength and even bone density. That's because their bodies are no longer subjected to the constant gravitational pressure, or stress, that is exerted upon them when they are on earth. Gravitational stress is a good thing when it comes to the health of your body. Lack of gravity and reduced gravity isn't.

This fact provides a clue as to what is really involved when stress causes disease. That's because, in the vast majority of cases, it is not physical stress that is at the heart of disease, but mental and emotional stress. One of the leading researchers in this area is Bruce Lipton, PhD. Dr. Lipton is a world famous cellular biologist and the author of *The Biology of Belief*. After spending decades investigating how and why stress causes illness, he coined the phrase "The New Biology" to replace modern medicine's fatalistic philosophy that health and illness is primarily a matter of fate shaped by one's genes.

According to Dr. Lipton, none of us are at the mercy of our genes. Although we may be born with genetic predispositions towards certain types of illnesses, Dr. Lipton states that it is actually our habitual thoughts and beliefs (along with what we are exposed to in our environment), not our genes, that have the most influence over whether we get sick or not. His view, which is increasingly coming to be shared by scientists and physicians in many areas of our health care system, is based on many years of scientific research.

To better understand how thoughts and beliefs can influence your health for good or bad, let's take a closer look at how the body is designed to protect itself from disease. Doubtless you are familiar with the body's immune system. Doctors and patients alike consider the immune system to be the human body's first line of defense against disease. Its task is to identify invading microorganisms (bacteria, fungi, parasites, and viruses) and to attack and eliminate them before they can cause harm to the body's cells, tissues, and organs.

Important as the immune system is to good health, however, there is another body system that is equally as, and perhaps even more, important. This system is known as the hypothalamus-pituitary-adrenal (HPA) axis. The purpose of the HPA axis is to spring into action at the first sign of any external threats that the body may face. When there aren't any threats, the HPA axis is in what might be described as "idle mode." This state of idleness allows the rest of your body to flourish the way that nature intended. But when the hypothalamus center in the brain perceives an outside threat, it signals the HPA axis to "roll out" and do its job. This is known as the "flight or fight" response.

As soon as this signal is given, your body's adrenal glands increase their production of cortisol and other stress hormones, releasing them into the blood stream. Once this happens, blood vessels that supply oxygen and nutrients to your body's cells and organs are constricted so that more blood can be made available to nourish the tissues of your body's arms and legs, since it is primarily these extremities that the body uses to fend off external attacks and get out of harm's way. Prior to this response, the blood in the body is concentrated in what are known as the visceral organs. These are the organs responsible for digestion and absorption of foods and nutrients, excretion, and various other functions that provide for proper cell growth and production of cellular energy. As blood is rushed to the tissues of the arms and legs, the visceral organs, such as the stomach, kidneys, and liver, cannot function at 100 percent, causing all growth-related activities in the body to become limited.

As you can imagine, if this process continues for sustained periods of time, your body's overall functioning will start to suffer. But this situation is further compounded by the impact sustained "flight or fight" responses have on the immune system. During "flight or fight" responses, the HPA axis causes the adrenal glands to suppress immune function in order to conserve the body's energy reserves via the adrenals increased production of stress hormones. Stress hormones are so effective at suppressing immune function that the stress hormone cortisol in the form of cortisone or prednisone drugs are actually administered to patients who receive organ transplants to prevent their bodies' immune systems from rejecting the organs.

In humanity's ancient past, the "flight or fight" response played an essential role in helping to keep our ancestors alive in the face of such dangers as attacking animals and natural occurrences such as earthquakes, floods, and volcanic eruptions. Today, however, most of us are not faced with such physical dangers, and even when we are, they are usually short-lived events. However, PNI researchers have discovered that actual physical danger is not necessary to trigger the "flight or fight" response. It can also be triggered by your thoughts and beliefs. Simply put, if you habitually focus on thoughts and beliefs of a limiting or negative nature, you are causing your body to act as if it is in danger. Though the adrenaline rush that occurs in the face of an actual physical threat usually doesn't result, the "flight or fight response" still takes place. Additionally, it does so for long periods of time. This results in chronic production of stress hormones, resulting in chronic suppression of immune function.

Here is what Dr. Lipton has to say about this matter: "In today's world, most of the stresses we are experiencing are not in the form of acute, concrete 'threats' that we can easily identify, respond to, and move on. We are constantly besieged by multitudes of irresolvable worries about our personal lives, our jobs, and our war-torn global community. Such worries do not threaten our immediate survival, but they nevertheless can activate the HPA axis, resulting in chronically elevated stress hormones."

Chronically elevated stress hormones results in a chronically suppressed immune function, leading to a greater susceptibility to infectious disease. Additionally, because of how the visceral organs are also negatively impacted by chronic stress, many of your body's functions are also suppressed, setting the stage for impaired digestion, increased muscle tension, and eventual declines in cell and tissue function, which can lead to a wide range of diseases, including heart attack and cancer, *see* inset on page 151. (Unmanaged stress can not only cause cancer, it has also been shown to accelerate the growth and spread of cancer cells.) In addition to heart disease and cancer, stress is also a major risk factor for gastrointestinal disorders, skin problems, neurological and emotional disorders, and a variety of conditions related to immune dysfunction, ranging from the common cold to arthritis, herpes, and even AIDS.

Recently, researchers in Sweden discovered that chronic stress incurred by middle-aged people can also play a major role in triggering the onset of Alzheimer's disease and dementia decades later. Most likely this occurs because of the way chronic stress, through its effects of various hormones, can negatively impact the brain.

Finally, with regard to maintaining acid-alkaline balance, stress also makes your body more acidic. Magnesium is one of the primary minerals your body uses to buffer that acid. Therefore, stress causes you to deplete magnesium faster to neutralize the acid. During times of fleeting stress, this may not be problematic, but since chronic stress is hardly rare these days, it becomes a major drain of magnesium. This, in turn, makes it increasingly difficult for your body to maintain its proper pH levels.

Based on these facts it's clear that one of the most important steps you can take to ensure your health is to deal with stress effectively. To effectively do so, you first must become better aware of the types of stress to which you are most commonly exposed.

POTENTIAL SOURCES OF STRESS IN YOUR LIFE

There are various types of stress and each of them has associated triggers. By knowing them and understanding their causes, you can more effectively ward off their stressful effects before they become chronic. The most common types of stress include:

- emotional stress
- environmental stress
- physical stress
- social stress
- spiritual stress

Emotional stress. Causes include suppressed or inappropriately expressed emotions, such as anger, anxiety, depression, fear, and guilt; divorce or other breakups; death; suffering on the part of those you care for; chronic illness (yours or someone you love); lack of nurturing relationships/friends; and unresolved life issues from the past.

Environmental stress. Causes include exposure to allergens, chemicals and other environmental toxins; fluorescent lights; computer and computer printers; cell phones; and household appliances.

Physical stress. Common causes include allergens, temperature (too hot or too cold), physical inactivity, illness, physical pain or trauma, and lack of sleep.

Social stress. Causes may include relationship issues with a spouse or significant other, family members and friends; issues with co-workers; unpleasant neighbors; job promotions or demotions; financial issues; and politics.

Spiritual stress. Causes may include not knowing your life's purpose, fear of death and/or the afterlife, lack of faith, and a variety of other existential issues, all of which can cause or worsen a spiritual crisis.

Take a moment to write down each of the above stress categories. Then list all of the particular stressors that affect you in each of these categories. Perform this exercise at a time when you know you won't be disturbed and take your time. Do the best you can to make sure each list is as complete as possible. Once you finish writing down your lists of stressors, go back to each list and rank each stressor on a scale of 1 to 10, with 1 being least stressful and 10 being most stressful. This exercise will show you the particular stressors that are currently causing the most problems for you.

If your stress index includes exposure to allergens, chemicals, or other environmental toxins, do what you can to limit your exposure to them. In addition, if environmental stressors *are* affecting you, I recommend that you consult with a health practitioner trained in environmental medicine. You can find out more about environmental medicine and find doctors who are trained in its practice by contacting the American Academy of Environmental Medicine (AAEM) at www.aaemonline.org. Similarly, if you are suffering from illness or physical trauma, consult with a physician if you are not already doing so.

DISTORTED THINKING PATTERNS

As with so many other things in life, when it comes to stress, it's often not the events that occur in your life that cause stress, it's how you *react* to those events. Many times, the events, by themselves, are neutral. For example, although nobody likes the thought of being stuck in traffic, that doesn't mean getting stuck in a traffic jam needs to be stressful. Although the most common reactions to traffic jams *are* stress-producing—such as anger, frustration, impatience, and tension—many people react to such situations calmly. Some even recognize it as an opportunity to devote their time positively doing something constructive, such as planning out their activities for later in the day.

Based on the above example, you can understand how people react to potential stressors in their lives is largely due to how they *think* about them. Many stressors aren't stressors at all, including traffic jams. They are simply neutral events. How you think about them determines whether or not they will cause stress in your life. Simply put, your thoughts can create or exacerbate stress in your life. By changing your attitude related to your thoughts, you can reduce or eliminate stress.

Thoughts that cause stress are usually a form of what psychologists refer to as *distorted thinking*. This means seeing things not as they are, but as we *choose to think they are*. Continuing with our example above, a traffic jam is simply that—a traffic jam. Of itself, it is neither "good" nor "bad," and has no power over you beyond preventing you from reaching your destination as quickly as you may wish. But if you think a traffic jam is a reason to become stressed and upset, then most likely stress and being upset is exactly what you will experience the next time you find yourself stuck in traffic. Whereas, if you think traffics jams are just minor inconveniences, then it is very likely that whenever you experience one, you won't be stressed by it.

By recognizing the role that your thoughts play in determining your reactions to what you experience in your life, you can understand why learning to consciously choose your thoughts can make a big difference in the degree to which stress affects you. In order to effectively do so, however, it's important that you first become aware of any distorted thinking patterns that you may be affected by. Doing so means knowing what types of distorted thinking patterns exist.

- **Blameful thinking.** People who think from a blameful perspective hold themselves or others responsible for every problem that comes their way, even when neither they nor others are to blame. Usually, blame also prevents them from moving on from past situations, and can also result in an inability to take responsibility for their present experiences.

- **Emotional reasoning.** This distorted thinking pattern is characterized by a belief that whatever you feel must be true. While feelings certainly can be valuable clues to what is true in our lives, automatically accepting your feelings as true is not always advisable. Here's an example of how emotional reasoning works. Let's say you are in a conversation with a handful of people and say something that you instantly regret because it made you appear uninformed. As a result, you may feel stupid. Under normal circumstances, such a feeling is understandable but is not apt to last. In fact, you might find yourself laughing at your temporary show of ignorance and never think about it again. But people affected by emotional reasoning will most likely react differently. As a result of momentarily feeling stupid, they are likely to start believing that they *are* stupid, despite all evidence to the contrary. Another example of emotional reasoning is equating making a mistake with the belief,

"I never get anything right." Again, a temporary feeling was transformed into an unexamined, ongoing belief. Such beliefs and thoughts about yourself can be very stressful. Ironically, these beliefs and thoughts aren't even true!

- **Negative thinking.** Negative thinking involves focusing on the negative details related to the events and people we encounter, to the point where all positive details are filtered out. This leads to a distorted magnification of the negative details, making them worse than they actually are. People who are negative thinkers tend to willfully refuse to see "the bright side" of people or events. Such thinking can create and perpetuate stress.

- **Personalization.** This type of distorted thinking is characterized by the belief that everything people do or say is some kind of reaction to you. People who think in this manner take everything personally, perceiving slights, insults, and other negative intentions from people even when that is not the case at all.

- **Polarized thinking.** This type of distorted thinking is characterized by seeing things in "absolutes." People whose thinking is polarized tend to see things as "black or white," "good or bad," "sinful or spiritual," and so forth. When polarized thinking is present, there are no "grey areas" and no middle ground. Polarized thinkers are usually unable to view anything and anyone without automatically deciding that events and people are "good" or "bad", and therefore stressful or not stressful, *regardless of objective reality.* Unfair as this can be to those people polarized thinkers determine are "bad," it is often even worse for the polarized thinkers themselves. Not only does polarized thinking prevent people from developing a broader, and therefore less stressful, perspective of the people and events they encounter in their daily lives, it can also make it very difficult for them to accept themselves without judgment. A common example of this is a tendency to try and be perfect in whatever the polarized thinker might do. Such an expectation is extremely unrealistic, yet is not seen to be so by polarized thinkers. Therefore, when they inevitably fail to achieve the perfection they are looking for, they may deem themselves failures. Such a self-judgment can be very stressful and is apt to last a long time, causing stress to become chronic.

- **"Should have" thinking.** People who think from a "should have" perspective tend to have a list of ironclad rules about how they and other people should act. People who break these rules anger them. Additionally, they feel guilty if they violate the rules themselves.

- **Victim thinking.** This type of thinking is common in people who view themselves as helpless when it comes to certain people or events. People who think in this way believe they have no control over what happens to them, when in fact they do. Victim thinking prevents them from recognizing their ability to take control of their lives.

All of these types of distorted thinking create "lose-lose" situations that can turn neutral, and even positive situations, and social interactions into stressful ones.

Now that you've read about distorted thinking patterns, take time to examine whether any of the above ways of thinking apply to you. Don't be alarmed if the answer is yes. In truth, all of us fall into these types of thinking patterns from time to time. What matters most is becoming conscious of when you do so, so that you can consciously choose to move out of them.

Once you have identified the distorted thinking patterns that you are prone to, review the list of stressors you created above (see *How Stressed Are You?* page 150). As you do so, ask yourself what patterns of distorted thinking might be involved in the stressors that are most common in your life. Then ask yourself if the stressors would have the same effects on you if the way you think about them wasn't distorted.

Take your time with this exercise and be honest with yourself as you go through it. If you are, you might be surprised to discover that at least some of your stressors on your list needn't be stressful at all.

REFRAMING DISTORTED THINKING PATTERNS
AND THE STRESSORS IN YOUR LIFE

The first step in effectively dealing with distorted thinking patterns is to realize that they are occurring. If you completed the exercises above, you've already begun that process. (If you haven't, stop reading now and go back and do them before continuing further.)

Now we're to show you how to take this process one step further using a powerful method known as reframing. Simply put, reframing is a process that will help you to see things in a different way than you have seen them in the past. More specifically, reframing helps to remove the judgments that are the principal causes of distorted thinking patterns. You can use reframing with any situation that throws you out of balance and causes stress, whether it's a relationship issue, work-related, or an unexpected event, such as the traffic jam we discussed yesterday.

There are three steps in reframing process you can use to eliminate or defuse distorted thinking patterns.

1. The first step is to simply recognize and admit to distorted thinking when you find yourself doing it. Then, instead of just automatically reacting to the situation that triggered it, no matter how charged or tense or uncomfortable you feel because of the situation, take a moment to notice how your thoughts are contributing to what you are feeling. Then recognize that you have a choice in how you are responding to the situation at hand. You can also take a few deep breaths to help yourself calm down and relax. This will leave you ready for step two.

2. As you contemplate the situation that is triggering your stress, take time to consider all the possible ways you can deal with it. Remember, you are not a victim of circumstance and you always have a choice in how you respond to whatever life brings you. Knowing that, look at each potential response that you come up with and ask yourself, "Which is most appropriate for me? Which one will get me closer to my goal? Which one best serves me and brings me peace of mind?" Then choose accordingly.

3. The third step is practice. Distorted thinking habits do not occur overnight. Usually they are ingrained, unconscious patterns that have been with us for most of our lives. Therefore, it is unrealistic to assume you can get rid of them without a bit of time and effort. This is why practice is so important. The more you practice consciously examining your thought patterns, the more you will develop the ability to choose how you want to think about—and therefore respond to—people and situations that in the past triggered stressful reactions within you. Awareness is the key.

Once again, take a look at the list of stressors you wrote down when performing the exercises above. Select a person or situation on your list that in the past has caused you a high degree of stress. Once you have made your selection, spend time writing down all of the possible ways in which you could have responded differently to that person or situation. Your aim should be to discover for yourself the response that best serves you and which leaves you with the least amount of stress.

Again, being honest with yourself is very important when performing this exercise. Since you don't have to share what you write with anyone but yourself, there is no reason for you to ignore all possible responses that occur to you. Nor is there a "right" or "wrong" way to do this exercise. (Thinking there is, is an example of polarized thinking, a type of distorted thinking that we discussed above.) Simply allow yourself to think of as many possible responses to the stressor you've selected as you can. By doing so, you will discover the solution to the stressor you've been looking for (even if you didn't know you were looking for it). After that, it's just a matter of practicing applying it so that the person or situation no longer affects you in the same way.

CREATING A STRESS-FREE LIFESTYLE

As with everything else in your life, the amount of stress you experience and how well you cope with it is largely due to your lifestyle choices (*see* How Stressed Are You? on page 150). What follow are simple, yet highly effective, lifestyle tips you can use to both reduce stress in your life and manage it better. By incorporating the following guidelines into your daily routine you will soon begin to feel and be more stress-free.

- Be sure to get enough sleep and try to go to bed at the same time each night. (For more about how to achieve deep, restful sleep, *see* Chapter 10.)

- Don't skip breakfast and be sure the foods you eat are healthy for you.

- Exercise for at least 30 minutes for a minimum of three days each week. (You will learn a lot more about how to most effectively exercise in Chapter 9.)

- Schedule your day so that you have free time to relax and spend with your loved ones.

- Find a hobby you enjoy and commit to pursuing it on a regular basis.

- Know what's most essential and important in your life and commit yourself to that instead of wasting time on matters that are unimportant.

- Identify your fears and worries and examine them objectively. In most cases, you will find doing so will make them far less significant and much more manageable.

- Set up your daily schedule so that you have plenty of time to devote to your daily tasks, instead of having to hurry to meet your responsibilities.

- Don't be afraid of compromising, especially about matters that aren't significant.

- Once you decide to do something, act on it as soon as possible. Hesitations about taking action can dramatically ramp up your stress levels.

- Cultivate laughter in your daily life and make a conscious effort to find the humor in things.

- Make a commitment to yourself and those you care about to be more loving.

- Avoid long periods of isolation, especially if you live alone. Seek out and enjoy your friends and loved ones.

- Regularly engage in relaxation exercises and/or meditation (*see* page 170).

- Avoid the use of alcohol, caffeine, and comfort foods when you do feel stress. Such things are unhealthy for you and serve only to numb your problems temporarily, not resolve them.

- Don't be afraid to discuss your situation with your family or friends, or to ask for help if you need it. Be assertive in the requests you make so that you are treated with respect and taken seriously by others. And keep in mind that everybody is stressed to some degree. Recognizing this fact makes it easier to realize that the stress you may be experiencing is far from unique. By sharing your issues with others you will likely discover answers to your problems from those who have also faced them. In turn, you may also be able to provide them with your own helpful insights. After all, we are all in this experience of life together.

From the above list, choose at least one item that you can do today and put it into practice. Then, try to incorporate at least one more item into your daily lifestyle every few days. Do this at your own pace, *but be sure to do it*. As you do so, over time you will find that you are increasingly living a less stressful lifestyle without needing to work at it. All that is required to do so is making the commitment to try each of the above guidelines that have relevance to you and then repeat them on a regular basis.

STRESS-REDUCING SELF-CARE METHODS

As with health in general, when it comes to stress you need to be proactive. Rather than allowing stress to build up and become chronic, when you find yourself experiencing stress in any form, take a moment to identify what is triggering it and then do your best to resolve it. The self-care techniques that follow can help you do so. Not only are they effective for banishing stress, they can also be used to prevent stress buildup in the first place.

Diet and Nutrition. Poor diet can cause stress and worsen symptoms of allergies (both food and environmental), anxiety, depression, and hyperactivity, all of which, in turn, can create additional feelings of stress, setting a vicious circle in motion. To combat stress, your diet needs to be free of all foods to which you may be allergic or sensitive, as well as food additives, sugar, sodas, and simple carbohydrates. Instead, emphasize the dietary recommendations we made in Chapter 4. Also be sure to eat a healthy breakfast. Skipping breakfast can add to stress levels by making you more tired and irritable.

During times of stress, also be sure to increase your intake of magnesium-rich foods, since magnesium is quickly depleted in times of stress and acts as a potent anti-stress nutrient. Such foods include nuts such as almonds, Brazil nuts, cashews, and walnuts; green leafy vegetables such as beet greens, kale, spinach, and Swiss chard; and grains such as barley, brown rice, millet, quinoa, and rice and wheat bran. Seaweed, especially kelp, is also very rich in magnesium, and can be used as a seasoning. Not surprisingly, most of these foods are also alkalizing when they are digested.

Also be sure to drink plenty of pure, filtered water throughout the day, and minimize your alcohol intake to no more than one glass of red wine or beer per day. You should also limit your caffeine intake, since too much caffeine can over-stimulate you, leaving you feeling "wired" and more susceptible to stress. If you drink coffee, try to keep your daily intake to no more than two cups per day. Or you can substitute green tea, instead. Although green tea also contains caffeine, the amount it contains is much less than coffee. Additionally, green tea is rich in healthy compounds, including L-theanine, an amino acid, and *epigallocatechin gallate,* an antioxidant, both of which can help lower stress hormones.

In many cultures around the world, "tea time" is a daily ritual that is regarded as a time of rest and relaxation. Simply making the time to drink a cup of tea can act as an antidote to life's daily stressors. For best results, get in the habit of drinking 2 to 3 cups of green tea every day, and reach for a cup the next time you feel stressed. Or, if you prefer, relax with various other types of herbal teas. Other good tea choices include chamomile, peppermint, and valerian root, which is also an excellent aid for a good night's sleep.

The following nutrients can further improve your ability to cope with stress: vitamin A, B-complex vitamins, vitamin B6, vitamin B12, vitamin C, vitamin E, and magnesium. Essential fatty acids (EFAs) are also important, especially omega-3 oils. If you suffer from hypoglycemia, add chromium and the amino acid glutamine (take 1000 mg three times per day, half an hour before each meal).

Get a Massage. Receiving a massage one or more times each month has been shown to not only relieve stress but to also significantly enhance immune function. Self-massage is also quite valuable and can be easily learned. Forms such as acupressure and shiatsu massage or reflexology (massaging the hands and feet) are particularly valuable. Many instruction books on these subjects are readily available at any good book store.

Massaging your spouse or partner and being massaged is in return is a wonderful way to relieve stress, and can also enhance lovemaking and deepen your connection with each other.

■ **NOTE:** In choosing a professional massage therapist, make sure that he or she is reputable and certified. Ask to see such certification if you are unsure. A refusal on their part is a sure sign that you should take your business elsewhere.

Keep a Journal. Another way of coping with stress is by keeping a stress journal. Keeping a journal has become an increasingly popular method for relieving stress, as well as for improving health in general. Research shows that regularly writing in a journal—a practice known as journaling—is a very effective way to become more aware of one's thoughts, emotions, and beliefs, as well as for providing insights and solutions to one's problems. Because of these benefits, journaling can reduce stress and improve mood. Studies have also shown that journaling can even improve immune function, thereby increasing resistance to infectious disease. When journaling is done on a regular basis it usually results in increased self-knowledge. In a very real sense, journaling can help you become your own therapist.

For years, studies have shown how effective journaling can be for managing and reducing stress. One of the most interesting of these studies was published in the *Journal of the American Medical Association (JAMA)* in 1999. In the study, test subjects suffering from chronic asthma and arthritis were asked to write about the most stressful events of their lives for 20 minutes for three consecutive days. Four months later, researchers found a significant improvement in lung function in the asthma subjects, and a noticeable reduction in the severity of symptoms of the subjects with arthritis; all after journaling about stressful events for only three days.

The reason journaling works, so well, as a form of stress relief is because of how effective it is for helping people to become better aware of their thoughts and beliefs, providing them with opportunities to recognize and change those that might be limiting them. Journaling can also help you to gain more control over how you think and feel, making it easier for you to be less reactive to your life experiences and enhancing your ability to be more creative and effective in dealing with them.

In addition, journaling is an excellent way for you to discharge emotions such as anger, especially if you usually have a difficult time expressing such emotions because you believe them to be negative. Keeping such emotions bottled up inside of you only adds to your stress levels, and can lead to other health problems over time. By expressing what you feel in a journal, you can let go of these emotions, free of judgments or criticism from others.

Journaling can also promote better sleep, especially in people who have trouble falling asleep due to worry or other upsets and concerns. By writing about the things that you are upset or concerned about before you go to bed, you can free yourself from such worries, making it easier to let them go and get the rest you need.

To begin journaling, spend 20 minutes writing down whatever comes to mind as you consider what is currently causing you concern or stress in your life. As you do so, allow yourself to express whatever emotions you have related to your situation, knowing that what you write is for you alone and it is not meant to be shared. Don't edit yourself as you write. Write down whatever comes up for you and don't be concerned about spelling or grammar. After you complete this exercise, notice how you feel. Most likely you will experience an improvement in your mood and emotions, and don't be surprised if you also feel energized.

If you think that journaling is something you will benefit from on an ongoing basis, here are some tips you can use to make it more effective.

- Choose a specific notebook for your journal and use it only for this task.

- Spend 20 to 30 minutes every afternoon or evening writing in your journal, expressing whatever comes up for you.

- List whatever issues you are concerned with on the left side of the page.

- Think about what you can do to help resolve these issues and write down whatever solutions and insights occur to you on the right side of the page.

- Once you are done writing for the day, keep your journal out of sight.

- For best results, try to write in your journal at the same time each day. Doing so will make it easier for you to develop the habit of journaling.

Laugh Your Troubles Away. No doubt you've heard the phrase "Laughter is the best medicine." It turns out there is quite a lot of truth to that statement. Scientific studies have shown that genuine laughter reduces stress and the production of stress-related hormones while simultaneously boosting immune function. Laughter also provides us with what psychologists call "cognitive control," a term used to describe being able to influence how we respond to external events. Although the events themselves may be beyond your control, as you learned above, you do have a choice as to how you respond to them. Laughter enables you to shift the perspective from which you perceive such events so that they become less stressful and even humorous.

Learning to find humor in the situations you experience each day, and being able to laugh about them, can be powerful antidotes to stress. Your sense of humor provides you with the ability to find delight, experience joy and happiness, and release tension. Additionally, being able to laugh at a situation, problem, and even yourself, can be very empowering. That's why more and more physicians, psychologists, and other health practitioners regard laughter as a very effective self-care tool. People who regularly experience laughter each day tend to have more positive and hopeful attitudes and are far less likely to succumb to depression and worry, compared to people who don't laugh a lot.

Here are some tips to help you find more reasons to laugh, both by yourself and, if appropriate, with others.

- Increase your exposure to humorous materials.

- Build a "laughter library" by compiling humorous movies, TV shows, and comedy shows that you can watch whenever you feel a need to lighten your mood. Fortunately, due to the Internet, you can find many online versions of these items for free.

- Learn to stay in touch with the playful, childlike nature that all of us have within ourselves, but which can quickly get overlooked due to our daily life challenges.

- Spend time around happy people. Research shows that doing so can increase your own level of happiness. Happy people also tend to be prone to laughter, so spending time with them is apt to make you laugh more too.

- Focus on genuine laughter, not laughter at another's expense or laughter that is born out of cynicism. Laughter that is genuine is usually also spontaneous, which is the most powerful type of laughter when it comes to banishing stress and tension.

- Finally, make it a point to have fun on a regular basis by spending time each day doing something you enjoy and/or being in the company of people who make you feel happy. The more you do so, the more likely it is that you will find yourself laughing.

Listen to Music. Numerous studies have shown that listening to music you enjoy can banish stressful feelings within minutes. Ideally, choose music of a relaxed tempo and listen to it while lying down with your eyes closed. The effect physiologically can be very similar to meditation. However, if your stress is related to issues attached to anger or other strong emotions, you may find it more useful to listen to music that is more "aggressive" in nature, such as your favorite rock anthem. Music with a strong percussive beat can also be helpful, as it lends itself to dance movements. Don't be afraid to engage in such movements by yourself. Just a few minutes of doing so can often be all that is needed to jumpstart a more positive, energized frame of mind.

Meditate Stress Away. Meditation is perhaps the world's oldest method for dealing with stress, as well as for providing a wealth of other significant benefits. Meditation has been an integral part of spiritual disciplines in both the East and West for thousands of years. Since the 1960s, meditation practices have also been extensively researched by Western scientists. Since that time, a very large body of research has found that meditation, when practiced regularly (once or twice a day), provides numerous health benefits of both a physical and psychological nature. Studies have shown that meditation results in a reduction of many of the physiological and biochemical markers associated with stress, such as decreased heart rate, decreased respiration rate, and improved regulation of stress hormones such as cortisol. In addition, meditation has been shown to increase brain waves associated with relaxation.

In its simplest form, meditation can be defined as any activity that keeps your attention pleasantly anchored in the present moment. In this state, your mind becomes calm and focused, and less apt to react to memories of the past or concerns about the future, both of which are major sources of chronic stress that can negatively impact your health.

The simplest form of meditation involves sitting quietly and focusing your attention on your breath (for more on the health benefits of breathing, see Chapter 7). When you are stressed, anxious, agitated, distracted, frightened, or otherwise upset, your breathing rate will tend to be shallow, rapid, or uneven. But when your mind is calm and focused, your breath becomes slow, deep, and regular. Regular practice of meditation leads to improved respiration rates, which in turn provides the health benefits listed above. Additionally, research has shown that the more people meditate, the more resistant they become to reactive behaviors and thought patterns that can cause stress and impair health. Long-term practitioners of meditations also tend to be calmer, happier, and more energetic than they were before they learned to meditate.

Wouldn't you like to enjoy such benefits? You can begin to do so by practicing the following meditation exercise for 15 to 20 minutes once or twice a day.

- Find a quiet place where you will not be disturbed and sit comfortably in a chair. Keep your spine straight and relax your shoulders, letting them drop slightly.

- Close your eyes and bring your attention to your belly as you breathe in and out in a relaxed manner through your diaphragm. Notice your belly gently rise as you inhale and descend as you exhale.

- Keep your attention focused on your breathing. At first, this may be difficult to do. If so, don't worry. Each time you notice that your mind has "wandered off" simply notice the thoughts that took your attention away from your breath and then return your focus to your belly and the rhythm of your breathing. No matter how many times you find your attention wandering— and you can be sure it will, especially at the beginning—simply bring it back to your breath. As you do so, you will eventually start to perceive how your thoughts flow by you, like leaves carried away on a stream. Instead of becoming absorbed by your thoughts, increasingly you will find yourself simply witnessing them from a calm state of detachment.

Ideally, you should practice this exercise twice a day, but once a day is fine, at first, if that is all the time you can spare. For best results, try to meditate at the same time each day, whether you feel like doing so or not. Practice this meditation exercise for at least one week, and then notice any changes in how you feel and act as a result.

Sex. Making love to someone you genuinely care about is not only a powerful way to relieve stress, it is also one of the deepest forms of human communication, and can have tremendous healing effects when not engaged in obsessively.

Showers and Baths. Water has an amazing capacity to heal. Taking a shower upon arriving home can quickly dispel any upsets brought home from work. And a soothing hot bath before retiring has been touted for its healing effects in Asia for centuries. Until the advent of modern day plumbing, baths were considered a luxury. Now they are a luxury all of us can make use of on a daily basis.

Take a Break. The following recommendation is particularly useful for people who sit at a desk during most of their working day. Once an hour, for no more than a minute or two, step away from your desk and take a stretch break. Exaggerate a yawn and feel your body really stretching comfortably. If you can, duck outside

Beating Stress by Listening to Your Heart

No doubt, you are aware that your heart is directly involved in all of the emotions you experience. You probably also know that emotions such as anxiety, fright, and stress can increase your heart rate. A "pounding" heart rate is almost always found during times of strong emotions. But scientists have found that even the slightest change in emotion can immediately change heart rhythm (the rate your heart beats).

Contrary to popular belief, a healthy heart does not beat at the same steady rate throughout the day. Heart beat rates vary, even during sleep. And the change in heart beat rhythm is now recognized by scientists as a communication tool that signals messages to and from the heart, brain and body.

Much of the recent research in heart beat rhythms and their relation to stress has been conducted by scientists at the Institute of HeartMath®, in Boulder Creek, California. For over 18 years, researchers there have explored the heart's "intelligence," and developed a variety of techniques, including the one on page 174, for using that intelligence to dramatically reduce stress. These techniques have been clinically proven to turn off the stress response and lower the release of cortisol, improve mood and cognitive performance, and reduce high blood pressure and the risk of dying from heart disease. The research conducted at the Institute of HeartMath conclusively shows that when people learn how to modulate their heart rate variability, they can quickly and effectively reduce negative reactions to stress and improve their overall health.

One of the most popular techniques developed by HeartMath researchers is known as the *Freeze-Frame*. It will enable you to stop your stress response to difficult situations by replacing negative perceptions with positive feelings, such as appreciation, enjoyment, and love. Research shows that these positive emotions restore calm and control to the heart rate.

Here are the five steps you can use to practice the Freeze-Frame technique the next time you find yourself in a stressful situation.

1. As soon as you recognize your stressful feeling, take a "time out" and "freeze" it.

2. Make a sincere effort to shift your focus away from whatever racing thoughts or upset emotions you may have, placing your focus instead on the area around your heart. Imagine that you are literally breathing through your heart to help focus your energy in this area. Do this for at least ten seconds.

3. Now recall a positive, enjoyable feeling or memory that you've had in your life and allow yourself to re-experience it.

4. As your renewed experience of the positive feeling you've selected takes hold of you, mentally ask your heart: What would be the best response to the situation I am in, that would take away my stress and minimize the return of stress in my future?

5. Listen to the response your heart provides and act on it.

This deceptively simple process can quickly rein in your reactive mind and emotions to help you find the most effective and appropriate response to your situation. But you don't have to wait for stress to strike before you practice the Freeze-Frame technique. You can practice it anytime. Doing so will help you become aware of your heart's intelligence, and over time deepen your connection to heart-centered emotions such as calm, peace, love, and happiness.

To find out more about the Institute of HeartMath and the research they've conducted, visit www.heartmath.org.

for a breath of fresh air as well. Instead of interfering with your deadlines, you'll find this simple routine will actually produce more energy and make you more productive.

Another useful technique for computer users, which can also help eyestrain, is to periodically cup both eyes with the palms of your hands. Take a few deep breaths and focus on the soothing energy of your hands moving into your eyes and down through your body. This is a wonderful pick-me-up to try three or four times during the day.

Take a Deep Breath. Breathing is one of the easiest stress-release methods available to all of us. The next time you notice that you are stressed or feeling tension in your body, close your eyes for a few moments and allow yourself to take ten deep breaths. Don't force them. Breathe in through the belly, inhale as fully as you comfortably can, then let the exhale naturally follow. Learning to do this on a regular basis throughout the day can pay big dividends and keep stress well at bay.

Take a Nap. Thomas Edison was one of the most creative and productive individuals the world has ever known, and he was famous for taking short naps throughout the day. Not only did he commonly exhibit far more energy and endurance than most of his employees, he also claimed that his naps led to the dreams that were the source of many of his greatest inventions, including the light bulb. While napping may not be possible while at work, making time to lie down for ten or twenty minutes after you arrive home can prove extremely refreshing and a wonderfully relaxing antidote to stress.

Walk Away from Stress. Physical exercise is another excellent means of reducing stress, so long as you do not overdo it. You will learn quite a bit about how to create a healthy exercise program for yourself in the next chapter. For now, we want to share with you one of the easiest and most effective exercises you can use to release stress: Go for a walk.

Besides being one of the most effective ways to exercise, walking can also be very relaxing. In addition, many people who regularly take walks find that it helps them to come up with new solutions to their challenges and problems.

We encourage you to try to walk every day for 20 to 30 minutes, starting today. If you are not used to regular exercise, start slowly, at first walking no more than once around your block. The point is to make walking a part of your daily routine and to keep at it until you can comfortably walk 20 to 30 minutes at a time.

SOCIAL CONNECTIONS AND STRESS RELIEF

One of the most enjoyable and effective ways for reducing and managing stress is by regularly spending time with people whose company you enjoy, especially your spouse or partner, other family members, or your best friend. Research has consistently shown that people who have strong relationships with others are far less prone to illness than people who primarily live lives of solitude. People with strong social connections also tend to live longer than people who are loners, and to cope better with whatever challenges life may bring their way. In fact, based on a growing number of studies about social connections, researchers now recognize that social isolation is statistically as dangerous as smoking, high blood pressure, high cholesterol, and lack of exercise.

Here are some of the reasons why strong connections with family and friends are so special—and so important.

Comfort. The people you love and who love you tend to be those you don't have to fill in the blanks with. They already know all the inner details of your life. It's like picking up a book and knowing exactly where you left off. You can cut to the chase and get right to the heart of any discussion because all the background information has already been stored away.

Connectedness. One of our most basic fears is being alone. Whether your best loved ones are nearby or in another time zone, just knowing they are there provides comfort. It gives you a sense of being connected and not just free-floating in space. So if you find yourself feeling isolated, whether physically or emotionally, pick up the phone and call someone you love. Both of you will feel better for it.

Life Lessons. When a loved one does something you disagree with, you're more likely to confront them and discuss what has upset you than if it's a person you aren't as familiar with. Getting through this with someone with whom you are close helps to prepare you for other times in life where you will need to face a difficult situation.

Loyalty. Loyalty means never having to worry about someone spilling your secrets or talking about you behind your back. Loved ones equal built-in trust. Most likely, you've spent years building your bond, which just gets stronger over time. Your loved ones will be on your team no matter what. They will be honest with you, but won't betray you.

A Fresh Perspective. We are all individuals, with different experiences and opinions, but being able to share things with loved ones can help you learn new things about yourself. The things they share with you can open your eyes to new ideas and ways to think about the world around you. By bringing a fresh perspective to a problem, things have a better chance of changing. Loved ones can help you find those "A-ha!" moments that lead to solving problems.

Personal Growth. Having strong connections with people you love means sharing experiences. Sometimes, when we get stuck in our own routines, it's nice to hear about what other people are doing. Doing so can provide us with different perspectives on life, which can often lead to growth and new discoveries.

Self-Esteem Boost. Your loved ones also help you to develop your self-esteem. Having someone in your life who thinks you are important—someone who wants your opinion on things and who values your company—makes you feel wanted, boosting self-esteem.

Unconditional Support. Your loved ones have seen you at your best and worst, and they love you either way. It's important to have someone in your life with whom you feel totally at ease with.

If you find yourself in need of a good friend, remember that it is never too late to rekindle old friendships or to make new ones. All that is necessary is a willingness to take risks and make the effort. As you do so, you will start to find that your overall moods and feelings of contentment will automatically improve.

The next time you find yourself dealing with stress choose a loved one with whom you'd like to spend time and let him or her know. You can do this in person or through a phone call (try to avoid doing so through email). Share what's on your mind and let your loved one do the same thing. Before you know it, whatever cares you have will start to feel lighter.

Altering your social relationships in a positive manner cost you nothing. However it can add a great deal to the quality of your life. By utilizing any or all of the eight suggestions above, research has shown you can greatly reduce your stress levels.

CONCLUSION

Now that you've read this chapter, we hope you understand how vitally important it is that you do all you can to manage stress in your life. By making a commitment to incorporating at least some of the stress-busting methods we've shared with you, you will soon find yourself dealing more easily with stress whenever it arises, and also more resistant to stress in the first place. In turn, as your stress levels diminish, your levels of health will increase, as will positive feelings of contentment, joy, and accomplishment.

In the next chapter we will explore, in-depth, another part of the Acid-Alkaline Lifestyle that is also essential to your overall well-being—exercise.

9

If You Don't Use It,
You Will Definitely Lose It

No discussion of health can be complete without including the subject of exercise and physical activity. In this chapter we are going to provide you with the guidelines you need to create an exercise program that is tailored to your unique needs and requirements. First, though, let's examine why exercise is so important.

Regular and appropriate exercise is essential for good health, and for preventing and reversing most of the health problems afflicting our nation today. The human body is designed for daily physical activity. However, as a nation, we have become increasingly sedentary, which is one of the primary reasons we now face such a daunting health crisis in this country. This alarming trend is especially true of our children, 25 percent of whom are unhealthily overweight or obese.

Numerous studies show that sedentary people, on average, don't live as long or enjoy as good health as people who exercise regularly. Based on these studies, a growing number of researchers and physicians now believe that lack of exercise is a more significant risk factor for decreased life expectancy than the *combined risks* of cigarette smoking, high cholesterol, being overweight, and high blood pressure. The scientific evidence conclusively makes one fact very clear: *Being unfit means being unhealthy.*

Here is a breakdown of the many benefits that regular exercise and physical activity can provide:

- increased longevity

- prevention of heart disease, cancer, and other serious, degenerative diseases

- improved recovery from heart disease and reduced risk of repeat heart conditions

- prevention of and relief from tension

- decreased "fight or flight" response, and therefore less stress

- prevention of and relief from anxiety and depression

- reduced risk of alcoholism and drug addiction

- increased muscle to fat ratio, making dieting and weight loss easier

- increased muscular strength

- increased flexibility

- improves balance, especially among older people, and diminishes the risk of falls and injury

- better quality of sleep

- improved mental function

- increased stamina and energy

- increased aerobic capacity

- improved self-esteem and greater confidence

- increased incidence of positive attitudes and emotions, including joy

Regular exercise also aids digestion, increases circulation, stimulates the lymphatic system (your body's filtration and purification system), and promotes enhanced levels of positive emotions and balanced mood. (Regular exercise of an aerobic nature has been shown to increase serotonin levels in the brain. Serotonin levels are associated with feelings of calm and well-being, improved brain function, and enhanced sleep.) Given all of the above benefits, you can see why we so strongly recommend that you make regular exercise a priority in your life.

A HEALTHY EXERCISE PROGRAM

Now let's take a look at the three elements that a healthy exercise program needs to address: *aerobic capacity, muscle strength,* and *flexibility.* The recommendations that we will be providing you with consist of a blend of exercises and physical activities that will help you increase each of these three elements. They incorporate a blend of strength training, aerobic, and stretching exercises that work in conjunction with each other to provide you with everything you need to make exercising a primary self-care health tool in your life.

Strength Training

Building and maintaining muscle strength is an essential component of your overall exercise program. This is particularly true as you age. Research shows that strength training helps to maintain healthy hormone levels, improve metabolism, reduce the risk of bone loss, and improves your body's ability to efficiently burn calories.

Weight training (weight lifting and training on weight machines) is perhaps the most popular form of strength training, but you can get many of the same strength-building benefits without the use of such equipment. Moreover, not having to rely on weights and weight machines makes it far likelier that you will commit to your training routine. For that reason, the exercise program we have created for you does not require such equipment.

Aerobic Exercise

The word *aerobic* means *with oxygen.* Aerobic exercise refers to prolonged exercise that requires extra oxygen to supply energy to the muscles. In general, aerobic exercise causes moderate shortness of breath, perspiration, and an increase in resting pulse rate.

The primary beneficiary of aerobic exercise is the heart muscle, due to the increased oxygen that such exercise provides to it, as well as the rest of your body. Jogging, bicycling, running on treadmills, and using stair climbers are all popular forms of aerobic exercise, as are swimming and sports such as tennis, racquetball, and basketball. However, the easiest form of aerobic exercise is walking.

Until recently, it was thought that one had to walk an average of 60 minutes per day to get adequate aerobic benefits. Newer research, however, indicates that you can receive all of the benefits of a 60-minute brisk walk in only 15 to 20 minutes a day by varying the intensity of your pace. We explain how to do this on page 189.

Stretching

The final component of your exercise routine involves stretching, which helps to increase and maintain your body's flexibility. This is important because lack of flexibility can severely inhibit your physical performance, lead to poor posture, and increase your risk of injury. In addition, increased flexibility also leads to improved strength and function, allowing your body's muscle groups to operate at peak efficiency. Other benefits of flexibility include improved circulation and greater suppleness of your body's tendons, ligaments, and connective tissues.

There are a variety of exercises that improve flexibility, such as yoga, Tai chi, and various types of bodywork, such as Rolfing and the Feldenkrais Method, all of which are excellent. However, once again, we don't want you to have to rely working with practitioners of these methods. Rather, our goal is to provide you with all you need to be able to improve and maintain your body's flexibility on your own. Which is why we've created an easy-to-do, yet highly effective stretching program you can do at home and when you are traveling.

By combining exercises that provide all of the above benefits and performing them according to our recommendations, you will soon find yourself feeling healthier and more fit than you might believe is possible right now.

HOW TO MAKE YOUR EXERCISE ROUTINE WORK BEST FOR YOU

Now that you understand why regular exercise is so important, as well as the three essential elements that a proper exercise program needs to include, let's move on to some tips you can use to get the best results from the exercise program we are about to share with you. By following these guidelines, you can not only be assured of the best results, but can also be sure of being able to perform your exercise regimen without fear of injury or over-exertion.

■ **NOTE:** If you have an existing medical condition or are just starting to exercise, be sure to consult with your physician prior to beginning the program. Once your doctor has cleared you for exercise, be sure to abide by the following guidelines.

- Avoid exercising, especially aerobic exercises, during times of emotional crises or when you are angry. Exercise under such conditions is counter productive and can put a dangerous strain on your heart.

- Wait at least two hours after eating before exercising. Additionally, when exercising before meals, wait at least 30 minutes after your exercise session ends before eating. Also drink plenty of water at least half an hour before you begin. You can drink water during the exercise session, if you are thirsty, but do so sparingly.

- Breathe! When performing any type of exercise, be sure to breathe in a relaxed, deep manner. Doing so will add to the benefits of the exercise itself by increasing the amount of oxygen that is available for your body's cells, tissues, and organs.

- Adopt a positive attitude about exercise and make it fun. By focusing on the important health benefits that exercise provides, you will enable yourself to more easily achieve them. A positive mindset can also make exercise fun and more enjoyable. You are more likely to continue exercising if you are doing something that you like.

- Listen to music you enjoy. Listening to such music when your exercise can not only increase your enjoyment during your exercise routine but can also provide you with a soundtrack to enhance your pace and overall performance.

- Be sure to start off any work-out/exercise session with proper warm-up and stretching exercises. This will help to avoid post-exercise soreness or injury.

- Wear the proper attire when exercising, including shoes with the proper support for the activity. Tight clothing and shoes can restrict your circulation and dissipation of heat during exercise. Avoid them.

- If you exercise outdoors, be sure to dress appropriately for the weather.

- When exercising indoors, make sure your room is well ventilated. Open windows or turn on the fan or the air-conditioner during summer months to avoid exercising in a room that is too hot.

- Just as warming-up and stretching is important as you begin each exercise session, so is a cool-down period at the end of your exercise activity. This should include at least several minutes of gentle stretching or walking.

By following the above guidelines, you will be sure to get the most benefit from the exercises you perform. Ideally, your weekly exercise program should include a combination of aerobic, strength-training, and stretching exercises. What follow are the benefits that each category of exercise provides.

YOUR DO-IT-ANYWHERE, COMPLETE EXERCISE PROGRAM

The remainder of this chapter consists of recommendations that have been specially tailored to meet your specific, individualized needs. In addition, the exercises we've selected for you can be performed at any time, without the need for a gym membership or exercise equipment and are designed to easily fit into your overall daily routine. In other words, no excuses. You are perfectly capable of performing each of the exercises routines that follow. By doing so, you will soon begin to notice improvements in your health that will continue as long as you make exercise a part of your daily life.

STRETCHING EXERCISES

We recommend that you make stretching a daily part of your life. To understand why, consider what animals do immediately upon awaking each morning. That's right, they stretch. Morning stretches do not take long, yet set a positive tone for the rest of your day.

In addition to the morning stretch routine we've created for you, we have also created additional stretching routines that you can perform after strength training. (Recent scientific studies have found that stretching before strength training exercises can actually be harmful, whereas stretching done after strength training exercises are completed can enhance the overall benefits that strength training provides.)

■ *MORNING STRETCH ROUTINE*

Frequency: Every Day

Duration: 5 to 10 minutes

Do the following series of stretching exercises every morning soon after you get out of bed.

Neck bends. Stand or sit up straight, with your head, neck, and upper torso aligned. Without straining, inhale deeply. Then exhale, bring your head forward so that your chin tucks into your chest, stretching the muscles in the back of your neck. Once you complete your exhalation, inhale once more, lifting your head up and back so that you stretch the front muscles of your neck. As you bend your neck forward and backward, make sure that your shoulders do not move. Repeat this sequence three times.

Next, return to your original position, with your head facing straight. Inhale, then, as you exhale, turn your head as far to your left as you can without straining, bringing your chin in line with your shoulder. Inhale once more and return your head to its original position. Then exhale, this turning your head as far right as you can. Repeat the entire sequence three times.

Once you finish the second exercise above, return once more to your original position. Inhale, then, as you exhale, stretch your neck leftward, bringing your left ear as close as you can to your left shoulder without straining (don't move your shoulder). Inhale and come back to center. Exhale again, this time bringing your right ear as close as you can to your right shoulder. Repeat entire sequence three times.

Finish your neck bends by neck rolls. Begin by lowering your chin to your chest and then slowly rotating your head in a clockwise motion, inhaling as your head rises, and exhaling as you lower it, bringing your head forward and down. Do this three times. Then reverse the rotation, and rotate your head counterclockwise three times. Be sure to allow your head to rotate freely and loosely, without strain.

Shoulder lifts. Stand up straight with your arms hanging loosely at your sides. Without moving your head, inhale and slowly tense and lift your left shoulder up towards your left ear. Then exhale, relaxing your shoulder and letting it drop. Repeat three times. Do the same with your right shoulder. Then repeat this process with both shoulders at the same time for an additional three times.

Torso twists. Continue standing in a relaxed manner, with your arms loose at your sides. Place your feet shoulder-width apart and bend your knees slightly. Keeping your heading facing forward, inhale and as you do so twist your upper torso to the right. Exhale and twist to the left. Repeat this process back in forth for a total of 12 times, inhaling as you turn right and exhaling as you turn left. When you finish 12 twists, remain standing and breathe in a deep, relaxed manner.

Overhead stretch. Stand erect with your feet shoulder-width apart and your knees slightly bent. Inhale and as you do so raise your arms and stretch them above your head, bringing the palms of your hands together as if in prayer. Without straining, stretch towards the ceiling as high as you can. Exhale, and relax your arms completely, letting them drop to your sides. Do this six times.

Forward bend. Stand erect with your feet shoulder-width apart and your knees slightly bent. Inhale and raise your arms over your head. Exhale and bend forward, with your fingers pointing toward the floor. Don't strain. Feel the stretch in your back, shoulders, and the back of your legs. Repeat this sequence for a total of 12 times.

Congratulations. You've just completed your morning stretch routine.

■ POST-STRENGTH TRAINING STRETCHES
Frequency: To Be Performed at the Completion
   of Strength Training Exercises

Duration: 3 to 5 Reps for Each Stretch

For each of the following stretching exercises:

- hold the stretch position for a slow count to 10
- do not bounce or jerk about as you hold each stretch
- alternate each stretch from side to side (example: right triceps muscle, then left triceps muscle)
- repeat each stretch to 3 to 5 times

Triceps stretch. Stand up straight and relaxed. Bring your left elbow over your head, with your left forearm hanging down behind your neck. Place your right hand on your left elbow and as you exhale, gently yet firmly use your right hand to stretch your left elbow downwards. Alternate this stretch between your left and right side so that both your left and right triceps muscles are stretched 3 to 5 times each.

Biceps stretch. Stand up straight and relaxed. Place both of your arms behind your back and interlace the fingers of your hands together. As you exhale, pull your arms away from your body, keeping your elbows straight. Repeat 3 to 5 times.

Calf muscle stretch. Face a wall and place your hands on it. Place one leg behind the other. Bend the front leg at the knee, while the back leg remains straight, keeping both of your feet flat on the ground. As you bend, move your hips forward so that you stretch the calf muscles of your back leg. Repeat this process with both legs, stretching each calf muscle 5 times. (If outdoors, you can do this exercise leaning against a tree.)

Hamstring stretch. While standing, raise your left leg and rest it on the seat of a chair. Keeping the foot of your right leg flat on the ground, lean forward and try to touch the toes of your left foot, exhaling as you stretch forward. Hold the stretch for a few seconds as you continue breathing, then inhale and rise back up. Now do the same with your right leg resting on the chair. Do a total of 5 stretches for each leg.

Quadriceps stretch. Stand on one leg while bending your other leg at the knee, taking hold of its foot with your hand. Use your hand to pull your leg closer to your body, holding the stretch for a few seconds. Then repeat the process with your other leg. Stretch both legs 5 times. (If you have trouble balancing while standing on one leg, support yourself by placing your free hand on a wall.)

After you complete the above stretching exercises, spend a few more minutes walking about and breathing regularly to complete your cool-down.

AEROBIC/CARDIOVASCULAR EXERCISE

Walking has been called the ideal exercise because it not only provides many health benefits, but it is something that just about anyone can do. It is also one of the easiest forms of aerobic exercise. However, normal walking has one major drawback in today's busy world. In order to get significant aerobic benefit from walking, most people need to walk for at least 30 to 60 minutes per day, which is something many people have trouble finding the time to do.

■ WALKING AND HIIT (High Intensity Interval Training)

Frequency: 5 to 7 days/week

Duration: 15 to 20 minutes

More recently, scientists have found that walking an average of 10,000 steps per day is a good way to improve health. But again, how many people have the time to count how many steps they take each day, let alone actually take them? Sure, the counting process can be attended to by investing in a pedometer, but we promised you an exercise program that doesn't require any equipment. (That doesn't mean you can't use a pedometer. If you want to use one, by all means do so.)

We also promised you a program that doesn't require a major time commitment on your part. To that end, we are going to teach you how to attain health benefits from walking for only 15 to 20 minutes 5 to 7 times a week that are far superior to what most people achieve from walking an hour or more each day. The secret to doing so is known as *high intensity interval training*, or HIIT.

HIIT is a type of aerobic and cardiovascular exercise that is performed at intense intervals. It is so effective because of what happens when you make it a part of your exercise routine. Unlike normal exercise, in which the greatest expenditure of energy and burning of calories occurs during the exercise routine itself and then stops, when you perform HIIT exercises, your body will expend energy and continue to burn calories for the rest of the day. Research has shown that HIIT exercises results in a burn rate of calories that is up to *nine times higher* that regular aerobic exercise. Just as importantly, HIIT exercises have been shown to be one of the most effective ways to eliminate fat buildup around the abdomen (belly fat). Excess abdominal fat is a major health risk that has been linked to a greater risk of heart disease, certain types of cancer, diabetes, Alzheimer's disease, and other serious health problems. Regular walking, no matter how much of it that you do, is ineffective at eliminating abdominal fat.

Another major benefit of HIIT exercise is the superior intake of oxygen that it provides your body, compared to other forms of exercise. Increased oxygen intake results in improved and sustained energy levels and improved metabolism, and has also been linked to a reduced risk of heart disease, cancer, and other debilitating conditions.

Additionally, walking combined with HIIT prevents the loss of muscle mass that can occur over time from walking for long periods over time. Regular long bouts of walking places the body in what is known as a catabolic state. Prolonged catabolic states result in a loss of muscle mass, which is not at all what you want as part of your fitness goals.

Because of the many significant benefits HIIT has been scientifically shown to provide, HIIT exercises are now a staple type of exercise employed by an increasing number of fitness trainers. But you don't need a fitness trainer to help you get the benefits of HIIT. Instead, all you need to do is turn your daily walks into your own HIIT program. Here's how to do it.

When you go for your walks be sure to wear appropriate walking shoes or sneakers.

- Start out walking at your regular pace for one to three minutes. Then walk as fast as you can yourself for 30 to 60 seconds. Then return to your slower, regular pace of walking for another one to two minutes, and then walk as fast as you can for 30 to 60 more seconds. Keep alternating between these two paces for a total of six cycles (each cycle consists of one regular and then one accelerated walking pace). Most people can complete this whole cycle within 15 to 20 minutes and possibly sooner.

Initially, walk along a flat pathway. Overtime, as your endurance and ability to walk using HIIT increases, seek out pathways that have inclines to get an even better work out. But don't do this immediately. Build up to it, instead.

■ **NOTE:** If you find that performing six cycles of HIIT is too much for you initially, that's okay. Reduce the amount of HIIT walking you do to one or two cycles, and then slowly increase the amount of HIIT walking cycles until you reach six full cycles.

- Also, be sure *not* to combine HIIT walking with strength training exercises, as combining the two will put unnecessary strain on your body. If you perform HIIT walks in the morning, do your strength training exercises in the late afternoon or early evening, and vice versa.

- Once your finish your daily HIIT walking routine, be sure to replenish your body with fluids, drinking either pure, filtered water or a healthy sports drink that does not contain sugar, sweeteners, or other chemical additives.

- Finally, if you have a treadmill, you can obtain the same benefits of HIIT by using your treadmill's appropriate programs that vary the pace of your workout in a way that parallels the HIIT walking routine above.

■ *JUMPING JACKS*

Frequency: To Be Performed as a Warm Up Exercise
  Prior to Strength Training

Duration: 5 to 10 Minutes

Prior to performing strength training exercises, it's important that you first "warm up" your body. Doing so will improve the benefits you get from strength training.

One of the easiest ways to quickly warm up your body is by performing jumping jacks. Jumping jacks provide aerobic and cardiovascular benefits and are not difficult to do. Perform them for 5 to 10 minutes, and then move on to the first of your strength training exercises.

Bounce Your Way to Better Health

Is it possible to bounce your way to health? According to many health experts, it is. All that is required is regular time devoted to bouncing on a mini-trampoline, also known as a rebounder. Although our goal in this chapter is to provide you with a complete exercise program you can perform without equipment, we want you to consider rebounding because of its many health benefits and the fact that it can be a lot of fun.

Many people, after adding rebounding to their exercise program, report increased energy levels, along with improved muscle tone, trimmer waist lines, and a variety of other health benefits. All from simply bouncing up and down for 10 to 50 minutes a day, making rebounding the "lazy person's way to exercise."

How and Why Rebounding Works

The primary reason that rebounding is such an effective type of exercise capable of providing so many health benefits is the combination of gravity and weightlessness that occurs while jumping on the mini-trampoline. As you begin to rebound, gravity exerts itself, pulling you downward, but as you touch down on the trampoline pad, you are immediately sprung upward into a momentary state of weightlessness. Researchers estimate that during each downward-upward-downward motion between 2 to 4 G (for gravity) forces are exerted on your body. The end result of this is that your body reacts as if it's carrying a heavy weight. But no strain is involved since the effect is so fleeting. Nonetheless, the overall effect starts a cascade of physical benefits.

According to NASA scientists who have studied the physiological effects of regular rebounding exercise, the temporary exertion of G forces caused during the exercise stimulates the body's lymphatic system while optimizing both blood circulation and the ability of your body's soft tissues and muscles to receive and use oxygen.

The effects on the lymphatic system are particularly impressive. The lymphatic system acts as the body's filtration system, and is responsible for ridding the body of toxins, dead cells and other cellular debris, heavy metals, and harmful microorganisms such as bacteria, fungi, and viruses. In this capacity, the lymphatic system plays a key role in assisting the body's immune system.

All too often, however, the lymph system becomes congested and clogged, causing a toxic buildup of the above substances that can ultimately lead to disease, many of which are quite serious. Further compounding the likelihood of this happening is the fact that, unlike the body's circulatory system, for which the heart acts like a pump of the blood, the lymphatic system has no such pump to ensure proper lymph flow and thus needs to be stimulated by exercise. Research has shown that rebounding is without question the most effective means of achieving this stimulation, which in turn accelerates the body's ability to eliminate toxins, germs, and waste products. This, in turn, leads to improved immune function.

Researchers have identified as many as 30 health benefits provided by regular rebound exercise. They include: improved energy, strengthening of the heart muscle and overall cardiovascular system, improved circulation, reduced blood pressure, reduced cholesterol, increased production of red blood cells, improved oxygenation of cells and tissues (meaning cells and tissues receive more oxygen), increased respiration, improved metabolism, improved muscle strength and muscle tone, improved coordination, improved mental function, improved digestion and elimination, and reduced body fat.

Getting Started

Rebounding is easy to incorporate into your daily lifestyle, and the benefits it provides can be achieved in as little as five minutes a day. All you need is regular access to a mini-trampoline, which typically range in price from $99 to $300, and are often available at sporting goods stores. (They can also be ordered online. Do a search for the term "rebounding exercise.") When selecting a rebounder, be sure that it is sturdy (good models will support a 300-pound person) and stands low enough so that you will not hit your head on the ceiling as you bounce (units that stand 10 inches off the ground are a good choice). Also be sure that the trampoline pad is supported by sturdy springs that are not connected directly to the frame. This will ensure a better and gentler bouncing action.

Once you've acquired a rebounder, the next step is simply to use it. Because of how gentle rebounding is, it is a safe exercise for just about anyone, regardless of their age or condition. (Health benefits can even be achieved by bouncing while sitting on the edge of the rebounder.) Some models also come with a support bar that you can hold onto as you bounce. Once you're on it, just start bouncing. Initially, you may want to only do so for a few minutes, but as you get used to it, try to aim for at least 5 to 10 minutes per day. After a few weeks, most likely you'll find rebounding to be one of the most fun and effective forms of exercise you'll ever do. And because it only takes minutes a day, rebounding is especially ideal for people whose lives are simply too busy. Ten minutes a day on a rebounder can make a big difference. If you are so inclined, try it and see.

STRENGTH TRAINING

The final pillar of your weekly exercise is strength training. Once again, our goal in creating this exercise pillar for you was to provide you with strength training exercises you can do on your own at any time of the day, without the need for weights or other strength training equipment. The key to doing so is known as body weight training that uses your own weight to create resistance, thereby strengthening your muscles.

■ *FULL BODY STRENGTH TRAINING WORKOUT*

Frequency: 2 to 3 times/week

Duration: 20 to 30 minutes

What follows is a full body strength training workout that focuses on all the major muscle groups in your body. Perform this workout two to three days a week, allowing at least one day in between your strength training workouts to let you body fully recuperate. Before beginning, make sure to warm up with 5 or 10 minutes of light cardio (jumping jacks) and end your workout with the series of stretches on page 185.

■ **NOTE:** Consult with your physician before trying this workout if you have any injuries, illnesses, or other conditions.

Body weight training routine. Perform one set of each exercise, one after the other, with brief (one minute) rests between exercises. Start out by completing one circuit of all the exercises. As your strength and endurance increases, move on to doing two full circuits of all the exercises for a longer, more intense workout. Then, after a few more weeks, do three full circuits of the exercises.

Initially, try to take a full five seconds for each rep of each of the exercises. Eventually, you can slow down your repetitions by taking a full 10 seconds for each rep. As you do each exercise, focus your attention on the muscles you are working, and be sure to breathe.

Perform the exercises in the following sequence:

1. **Push-Ups (Muscle Groups: Arms, Chest, Back):** Lay on the floor, stomach down, with your legs extended. Place your hands on the floor, next to your body and slightly below your shoulders, with your fingers facing forward. Balance your body on the balls of your feet and push up from the floor using your hands, exhaling as you do so, until your arms are fully extended. Then inhale and slowly lower your body back down to the floor until your chest nearly touches the floor. Repeat for a total of 10 reps.

   If you are unable to do a traditional push-up, try doing them against a wall. With your feet shoulder-width apart, stand one foot away from the wall, with your hands close to your body and slightly below your shoulders. Inhale and lean forward into the wall, supporting your body with your arms and hands. Bring your chest as close to the wall as you can without touching it, then exhale and push yourself away from the wall. Repeat for a total of 10 reps (one circuit). Slowly work up to a total of 20 reps. Once you can do 20 reps easily, then see if you can progress to a traditional push-up.

2. **Squat Thrusts (Muscle Groups: Glutes, Thighs, Hamstrings, and Quadriceps):** Stand up straight, with your legs shoulder-width apart. Face forward, keeping your chin up and your back straight, and bring your arms out in front of you, fully extended. Inhale and slowly bend your knees, squatting down as if you were sitting on a chair. At the bottom of your squat, hold your position for one to two seconds, then exhale and push up from your legs to return to your starting position. Repeat for 10 to 15 reps to make one circuit.

   To ensure you are squatting deeply enough, stand in front of a chair as you perform this exercise. You should squat far enough down that your butt is hovering only an inch or two above the seat of the chair.

   This exercise is very beneficial for people who are out of shape or who are older. If you fall into either of these categories perform squat thrusts gradually, and slowly work your way up to the full set of reps advised above, taking care not to over-do it.

3. **Lunges (Muscle Groups: Glutes, Thighs, Hamstrings, Quadriceps, Calves):** Stand up straight, with your legs shoulder-width apart. Face forward, keeping your chin up and your back straight. Place your hands on your hips. As you inhale, step your right foot forward as if you were about to lunge, while sliding your left foot backward. Bend down so that your right knee is directly over the toes and at a 90-degree angle. Hold this position for one second and then, exhaling, use your right leg to push back to your starting position. Now repeat this process, placing your left leg forward. Alternate between both legs for a total of 10 reps each (one full circuit).

4. **Wall Sit (Muscle Groups: Glutes, Quadriceps, and Calves):** Stand about two feet away from a wall, with your feet shoulder-width apart. Lean your back completely against the wall, and then

slowly slide down the wall until your thighs are parallel to the ground. You are performing this exercise correctly if you form a right angle at your hips and your knees, your back is flat against the wall, and your heels are flat on the ground. Once in this position, hold it for 10 to 30 seconds (start with 10 and slowly increase to 30 over the course of a few weeks), then slide back up and resume your standing position. Rest for another 30 seconds, and then repeat the process two more times (one full circuit).

As you continue to perform this exercise in the days ahead, try to increase your hold position by five seconds each time, until you are able to hold your position for one to two minutes.

If at first you find this exercise too difficult to perform, try doing a modified wall sit instead. You can do this by sliding down the wall until your lower body forms a 45-degree angle, instead of a 90-degree (right angle). As your ability to perform the modified wall sit improves, move on to the complete wall sit when you feel ready.

■ **NOTE:** If you feel pain in your knee or kneecap when your perform wall sits, stop the exercise immediately and consult with your doctor.

5. **Calf Raises (Muscle Groups: Calves, Ankles, Toes):** Stand up straight with your feet shoulder-width apart. Place your hands on your hips, and raise yourself up onto your toes. Hold this position for ten seconds, then drop back down to the floor. Repeat for a total of 20 times (one full circuit).

   Once you can do this exercise comfortably for a total of three full circuits, try placing the front of your feet on a two-inch thick book, such as a phone book, and performing calf raises from that position.

6. **Abdominal Crunches (Muscle Group: Abdomen):** Lie on your back with your knees bent and your feet flat on the floor. Place your fingertips to the side of your head just behind your ears. Push your lower back into the floor flattening the arch. As you exhale, curl up slowly so both your shoulders lift off the floor a few

inches. Hold for a count of two and then slowly return to your start position. As you perform this sequence, be sure not to tuck your chin to your chest. Instead, keep your head up. Repeat this sequence for a total of 10 to 15 times (one full circuit).

7. **Reverse Crunch (Muscle Group: Abdomen):** This exercise, performed in conjunction with the abdominal crunch above, ensures that all of your abdominal muscles are strengthened and tone. To perform it lie on your back with your hands out to your sides, and bend your knees. As you inhale, bring your knees toward your head until your hips come up slightly off the floor (be sure not to rock as you do this). Hold for one second and then, exhaling, slowly return to your starting position. Repeat this sequence for a total of 10 to 15 times (one full circuit).

8. **Back Extensions (Muscle Groups: Back and Abs):** This exercise is excellent for strengthening the back muscles while also toning the abdomen. Lie face down on the floor and place your arms straight in front of you. Contract (tighten) your abdomen and keep your abdominal muscles contracted throughout the exercise. Without straining, raise your arms and legs off the ground a few inches. Hold this position for a count of five, and then lower your arms and feet back to the ground. Repeat this sequence for a total of 15 to 20 reps (one full circuit).

9. **Corpse Pose:** Once you are finished performing the above exercises, lie face up on the floor, with your arms and legs spread loosely, as if you were a corpse on the ground. Close your eyes and breathe deeply and fully in and of your belly for a few minutes. This yoga pose is an excellent way to both relax and recharge your body. When you are finished, open your eyes and gently stand up to perform the post-weight training stretching exercises we shared with you on page 187.

Once you are done stretching, drink a glass of water or a healthy sports drink, and have a small snack of a healthy, protein-rich food.

CONCLUSION

The above combinations of exercises (aerobic, stretching, and strength training) are all you need to do to gain the benefits that regular exercise provides. We recommend that you experiment with them and, if necessary, adapt them to your specific needs. The key to long-term success is to find exercise activities you enjoy and commit to them on a regular basis. If possible, exercise outdoors, as the combination of fresh air and bright sunshine will make your activities more enjoyable, and provide even greater health benefits. If you enjoy other pleasurable activities, such as hiking, bicycling, or swimming, we encourage you to do them regularly as well.

As you begin your exercise program, remember that it is important to not try to accomplish too much too soon. Slow and easy is the rule, not "No pain, no gain." As you begin your exercise program stay at your level for at least five to seven days before you increase your activity. This allows you to progress in a safe and effective manner without overtaxing your body.

As we have already mentioned, if you haven't exercised in a long time, be sure to get the advice of your physician first. You may even want to initially train with a fitness coach or other professional. Or you may find exercise becomes more enjoyable if you do it with a friend or family member. Over a period of weeks, as you make exercise a regular part of your daily life, you will find that you can achieve more and will begin to notice improved energy and endurance, as well as increased happiness and personal satisfaction. Don't be surprised if your sex life improves, too!

Now it's time to explore the final element of the Acid-Alkaline Lifestyle—a good night's sleep. To discover how to ensure deep, restful sleep, turn to the next chapter.

10

To Sleep,
Perchance to Heal

good night's sleep is one of the most important factors for achieving and maintaining optimal health. It's also often overlooked and, for tens of millions of Americans, very difficult to come by. In this chapter you will learn why sleep is so important to your health, discover how to create a healthy sleep environment, and be taught a variety of things you can do to enhance how well you sleep, including lifestyle choices you can make to enhance sleep and rejuvenation, and a variety of self-care techniques that will further improve your ability to get a good night's sleep.

WHY SLEEP IS SO IMPORTANT

The merits of a good night's sleep are much greater that many of us recognize. It is an essential part of our life, but many of us know very little about what a critical part it plays in our well-being. What follows are the most important reasons why sleep is important for overall health.

Helps keep your heart healthy. Your heart and cardiovascular system are constantly under pressure. That's just a fact of daily life. Sleep helps to reduce the levels of stress and inflammation in your body. High levels of 'inflammatory markers' are linked to heart attacks, heart disease, and strokes. Sleep can also help keep blood pressure and cholesterol levels (which play a role in heart disease) within healthy levels.

Helps to maintain healthy weight. One of the lesser known benefits of sleep is that it helps regulate the hormones that affect and control your appetite. Studies have shown that when your body is deprived of sleep, these normal hormone balances are interrupted and your appetite increases, especially for foods high in calories, such as fats and carbohydrates, including sweets. Researchers have now established that lack of sleep triggers unhealthy weight gain and is also a factor in type 2 diabetes, a common result of chronic obesity.

Helps to repair your body. During sleep your body produces extra protein molecules. These molecules help to mend and repair your body at a cellular level. This includes repairing damage caused by stress, pollutants, infection, too much sun exposure, and free radical damage caused by poor diet and other factors.

Improves immune function. During deep sleep your body releases potent immune-enhancing substances that strengthen your immune system function. Lack of sleep can impair proper immune function, increasing susceptibility to infection and common illnesses such as cold and flu, respiratory conditions, and other diseases. Healthy, deep sleep also allows your body to release a significant amount of growth hormone that boosts the immune system and aids in the growth and repair of the body.

Improves memory. As you sleep your brain has the opportunity to process, organize, and correlate memories and new experiences gained during the day. In addition, sleep leads to greater mental alertness and concentration, making it easier to process new skills and knowledge. Healthy sleep also acts as an excellent aid in protecting against moodiness, irritability, and other unhealthy emotions. Recent research also shows that sleep is essential for eliminating toxins in the brain, thus helping to maintain healthy cognitive function.

Reduces stress. A good night's sleep can lower blood pressure and the elevated levels of stress hormones which are a natural result of today's fast paced lifestyle. There are physical effects of stress, such as excess 'wear and tear' on your body, and an increase in the aging and degeneration of organs, cells, and other body parts. By reducing high levels of stress, sleep helps to reverse these effects and encourages a state of greater relaxation. In addition, by reducing stress, sleep helps your body to maintain its stores of alkalizing minerals, including magnesium, which is quickly depleted during times of stress.

Based on these facts, you can understand why sleep is so vital for your overall well-being. Despite the facts, it is estimated that over 70 million Americans have trouble getting a good night's sleep at least a few times each week. Additionally, each year in the United States businesses lose an estimated $70 to $100 billion due to lost productivity of workers directly due to lack of sleep. Far more alarming, 24,000 Americans die each year in motor vehicle accidents caused by lack of sleep. In addition, recent research has found that lack of sleep (as well as too much sleep) is a major risk factor for premature death due to the harmful health effects it causes.

Prior to the invention of the light bulb and electric lighting in homes, most Americans averaged nine hours of sleep each night. Today, especially during the work week, that number has been reduced to 6 or 7 hours of sleep for most Americans, and in some cases much less, especially among people who are middle-aged or older. Yet sleep researchers have found that, with few exceptions, most people require at least 7 to 8 hours of sleep each and every night. That should be your goal, as well.

CREATING AN OPTIMAL SLEEP ENVIRONMENT

Your bedroom may be an overlooked factor that is contributing to unhealthy sleep. Follow the guidelines and you can transform your bedroom into a more conducive sleep environment.

FACTORS THAT CAN INTERFERE WITH A GOOD NIGHT'S SLEEP

In order to improve your sleep, it's important that you first understand the factors that may be contributing to poor sleep so that you can address those that may be affecting you. As you read what follows, identify any of the factors that apply to you and apply the relevant action steps that address them.

Diet

Poor diet and/or poor eating habits, such as eating late in the evening, only a few hours before retiring, can often cause or exacerbate sleeping problems. This is especially true of the standard American diet, which is high in salt, sugars, simple and refined carbohydrates, unhealthy oils, and convenience, processed foods, and lacking in organic fresh fruits and vegetables.

Excessive alcohol and caffeine intake can also cause sleep problems. Alcohol can disrupt your body's circadian rhythms and interfere with healthy REM sleep, while caffeine is a known stimulant that can leave you feeling one edge and unable to properly relax, thus preventing and interfering with sleep. Caffeine, in particular, has been linked by researchers to insomnia, periodic limb movement in sleep, and restless legs syndrome.

Action Step. Assess your daily diet and determine if there are changes that you need to make to it based on the information above.

Drugs

Drugs, both legal and illegal, can be powerful disruptors of healthy sleep patterns. Illicit drugs create a toxic burden in the body that can interfere with the ability to get a good night's rest. Many illegal drugs, such as amphetamines and cocaine, also act as stimulants, making sleep difficult and significantly altering the body's natural circadian rhythms.

Legal medications, both prescription and over-the-counter, can similarly impair your ability to get a good night's sleep. These include beta-blockers, cold and cough medicines (they contain caffeine and synthetic stimulants such as ephedrine), oral contraceptives, synthetic hormones, and thyroid medicines. In addition, all drugs, whether legal or illegal, create a toxic burden on the liver and can impair other organ systems as well, making sleep more difficult.

Action Step. If you are using illegal drugs, stop. Get help if you need to. Otherwise, over time, poor sleep will be the least of your problems. If you are on medications prescribed by your doctor, discuss the possibility of reducing your medication doses and eventually eliminating at least some of your meds over time.

Food Allergies and Sensitivities

Food allergies and sensitivities can interfere with your ability to sleep peacefully and restfully and are a frequent cause of sleep disorders.

Among the ways that food allergies and sensitivities can cause or worsen sleeping problems are the hypoglycemia (low blood sugar) they can cause, as well as increased histamine production. Sugar and carbohydrate foods are frequent triggers of food allergies that cause drops in blood sugar levels. When this happens, the body compensates by producing spikes in insulin production. This creates an adrenal stress reaction that puts the body in a state of stimulation characterized by jittery feelings and tension.

During allergic food reactions, the body can also produce elevated levels of histamine in the brain, disrupting brain chemistry. This, in turn, can greatly affect your ability to get a good night's sleep, and can often result in insomnia.

The most common foods that produce allergies and sensitivities are caffeine, chocolate, corn, dairy products, eggs, wheat, and wheat products, as well as sugars and refined carbohydrates. Any food can potentially trigger such reactions, however. If you suffer from sleeping problems that are accompanied by fatigue during the day (especially upon awakening and throughout the morning) and/or frequent feelings of irritability, most likely your condition is being caused or exacerbated by food allergies or sensitivities.

Action Step. If you suspect that you suffer from food allergies, try eliminating the suspect foods above from your diet. Do this for one month and note any improvements to your sleep, health, and energy levels during that time. If problems persist, consider working with a food allergy specialist or a doctor trained in environmental medicine. You can locate such physicians by contacting the American Academy of Environmental Medicine at www.aaemonline.org.

Geopathic Stress

Geopathic stress refers to energy fields within the earth that are imbalanced and capable of disrupting the body's bio-electrical fields, and therefore the health of those who dwell near such areas. The most common sources of geopathic stress are geological fault lines and certain large mineral deposits and streams. Manmade devices, such as computers, electric blankets and clocks, and electrically heated waterbeds, as well as common electrical current of 60 cycle frequencies, can also cause geopathic stress, as can power lines and power generators, due the electromagnetic frequencies (EMFs) they emit.

Research has shown that natural geopathic stress zones beneath or near sleeping areas, as well as geopathic stress caused by manmade devices in the bedroom, can significantly affect a person's sleeping patterns, and can also cause or contribute to a wide range of other health problems, including cancer, depression, headaches, and migraines.

Action Step. To compensate for manmade sources of geopathic stress, follow the guidelines we share. (See *Creating An Optimal Sleep Environment* on page 203.)

Lack of Exercise

Lack of regular exercise typically results in chronic muscle tension and the buildup of stress in the body, which can make relaxing and falling asleep more difficult.

Action Step. Try to fit in at least 20 to 30 minutes of physical activity in your daily routine. For exercise tips, *see* Chapter 9.

Overstimulation Before You Go to Bed

Over-stimulating yourself before you go to bed can make falling asleep more difficult. There are a variety of ways in which you can over-stimulate yourself, including late night exercise, watching television, or working on your computer, including checking your email. All of these activities serve to stimulate brain function by generating "busy mode" beta wave activity. While beta wave activity is essential for problem-solving and dealing with many other issues during waking hours, quick and restful sleep can only occur when beta waves in the brain subside, giving way to the more relaxed states of alpha and theta waves. (A fourth type of brain wave, known as delta wave, occurs during deep, dreamless sleep.)

Action Step. To prevent overstimulation, get in the habit of spending the last 30 minutes of your day in "quiet time" activities, such as mediation, prayer, or other relaxing activities that you enjoy. Doing so on a regular basis will start to prime both your brain and body to more readily shift towards sleep as you let go of the cares of the day.

Psychological Factors

Various psychological factors, including unresolved anxiety, depression, despair fear, and grief, as well as positive emotions such as excitement and euphoria, can interfere with your ability to get a good night's sleep. Such psychological factors can cause imbalances in your biochemistry and, if prolonged, can also create various other disturbances, such as indigestion and other gastrointestinal problems that can keep you awake at night. In addition, such factors can also interfere with the brain's ability to properly produce nerve signals and the production of hormones such as melatonin and serotonin related to restful sleep. Chronic stress can also cause depletion of the adrenal glands, further aggravating sleep disorders.

Action Step. Make use of the stress-reduction techniques we shared in Chapter 8. For other unresolved and troubling psychological issues, consider working with a mental health specialist.

Smoking

Smoking, as well as secondhand exposure to cigarette smoke can interfere with healthy sleep because of the chemicals and nicotine cigarettes contain. Nicotine acts as a stimulant and can cause insomnia and other sleep disorders, while many of the other chemicals contained in cigarettes can create a toxic burden on the liver to further disturb healthy sleep patterns.

Action Step. Avoid exposure to secondhand smoke. If you smoke, get help so that you can quit.

Structural Imbalances

Structural imbalances in your body, such as muscle tension and/or a misaligned spine, can contribute to sleep disorders due to how such imbalances interfere with the flow of nerve signals to and from the brain. They can also keep you awake at night due to the pain they cause in the muscles and joints.

Action Step. To help resolve structural imbalances, consider adding a few minutes of gentle stretching exercises to your daily routine (see Chapter 9). For structural problems that you cannot resolve on your own, consider working with a massage therapist, bodyworker, chiropractor, or osteopathic physician.

Unhealthy Sleep Environment

The environment of your bedroom can have a major influence on the quality of your sleep. Bedrooms that are excessively cold, hot, or humid, or which have poor indoor air quality and ventilation, can make healthy sleep difficult, as can sleeping in rooms that let in light from windows or other rooms, as well as sleeping on mattresses that are too hard, soft, or otherwise uncomfortable.

Action Step. Follow the recommendations we share in the next section, *Creating an Optimal Sleep Environment.*

- Keep your bedroom clean and free of dust. This means cleaning your bedroom at least once a week and washing blankets, sheets, and pillow cases frequently as well. An unclean bedroom not only interferes with restful sleep, it also makes you more susceptible to infectious microorganisms and can negatively impact your respiratory system as you breathe in dust while you are sleeping. To further prevent dust build up consider using an air purifier in your home, and also be sure that the filters on your heat ducts are professionally examined at least once a year and replaced as necessary.

- Be sure to allow for a flow of fresh air throughout your bedroom as you sleep. You can do this easily by keeping at least one window of your bedroom slightly open as you sleep. Breathing fresh, oxygen-rich air when you go to bed will not only enhance the benefits of sleep itself but also make it easier for you to fall asleep.

- Sleep on a comfortable mattress. What makes a mattress comfortable is a subjective experience. Simply put, you will know what type of mattress is most comfortable for you when you experience it. Despite what the investment in a new mattress may mean, if your current mattress is uncomfortable you will find the cost of a new mattress that meets your specific needs well worth it.

- Be aware that you might be sensitive to the materials in your pillow, blankets, and sheets. As a general rule, cotton or wool blankets and sheets and feather pillows are healthier choices than the same items made from synthetic materials.

- Make sure that the temperature in your bedroom is kept at a comfortable level. Temperatures that are too hot or cold can significantly interfere with your ability to get a good night's sleep.

- Make your bedroom a place of sleep, not a place to watch television. If you have a TV in your bedroom, consider moving it to another room in your home. Watching TV in bed keeps your brain in active mode, making sleep more difficult to come by once you turn in for the night.

- In addition to removing a TV from your bedroom, if you have one there, also try to keep your bedroom free of other electrical appliances, such as stereos, cell phones, computer, and radios. Again, your bedroom should be a place of sleep, not an entertainment or work center. Moreover, a growing body of research indicates that sleeping in a room full of electrical appliances can interfere with healthy, restorative sleep because of the electromagnetic frequencies such devices emit, even when they are not in use.

- These frequencies can cause what is now recognized as electromagnetic pollution that can negatively impact your body on an energetic level, making sleep more difficult, and also devitalizing you by draining your body's own energy. At the very least, be sure to sleep at least eight feet away from all such devices if you feel you must have them in your bedroom, and also unplug them before you retire for the night. For best results, though, banish all such devices from your bedroom.

- Sleep in the dark. This means not only turning off your bedroom lights when you go to bed, but also making sure that curtains and shades are fully drawn as well to prevent outdoor light from entering your bedroom. Sleeping in complete darkness helps your body to produce the hormone melatonin, which is essential for healthy sleep, as well as many other functions in your body. (To learn more about melatonin *see* page 217.)

Take a look at your bedroom to see how well it meets the above guidelines. Then, if improvements need to be made, please be sure to make them.

SELF-CARE APPROACHES FOR BETTER SLEEP

In the remainder of this chapter we are doing to share a variety of proven self-care methods you can use to enhance the quality of

Improve Your Sleep by Understanding Your Body's Circadian Rhythms

Research shows that healthy sleep is in part dependent on your body's internal "body clock," which is influenced by what are known as circadian rhythms. The term *circadian* is Latin and means "around a day." Circadian rhythms tend to follow the same cycles and patterns of the sun during a 24-hour period, and influence the times of day when you feel most awake and alert, as well as those times when you feel tired or sleepy.

People who have healthy circadian rhythms have little trouble rising early in the day with lots of energy, and also tend to easily fall and remain asleep at night, usually retiring well before midnight. This was the normal waking and sleeping pattern of our ancestors. However, due to many factors of the modern world, especially the amount of time we spend inside under artificial light, it is much easier to disrupt the body's natural circadian rhythms. When this happens, healthy, restful sleep is disrupted and various other physical and psychological health disturbances are apt to occur.

Prior to indoor lighting in homes, few people suffered from disruptions in their circadian rhythms. Typically, they rose at dawn and went to bed soon after the sun went down. Recognizing the importance of such a following, the cycles of the sun, Benjamin Franklin wrote his famous dictum, "Early to bed, early to rise, make a man healthy, wealthy, and wise." Many famous and successful people throughout history have followed his advice, routinely going to bed by 10 o'clock and getting up by 6 AM. Such people also tend to remain healthy and live long lives.

Many people today follow only half of Franklin's advice. While they get up early for work, they all too often fail to get to bed until midnight or later, thus failing to get an adequate amount of sleep each night. Other people still aim for 7 or 8 hours of sleep, but still go to bed late only to rise out of bed late in the morning. As long as they continue to sleep 7 or 8 hours each night, these people assume they are meeting their body's sleep requirements.

As it turns out, however, they most likely are not. That's because research also shows that it's not only how much sleep you get each night that counts, it's also when you get it. Scientists are increasingly finding out that Ben Franklin was right in ways he himself likely did not know.

A growing body of research indicates that the best quality of sleep occurs for most people between the hours of 10 PM and 6 AM. The reason for this is that the human body seems to be designed to begin the repair mechanisms that occur during sleep at approximately 10 PM. By going to sleep later than that, you interfere with the start of these repairs, making them less efficient.

Beginning tonight, try to go to bed at 10 PM and get up at 6 PM. If you are not used to going to sleep so early, you may find doing so is initially difficult to achieve. Even so, try to abide by it for at least a week, so that you have time to notice whether it leads to improvements in your sleep and overall well-being. If, after a week, you still find this "early to bed, early to rise" schedule doesn't suit you, try going to bed a bit later (10:30 or 11 PM), just so long as you are still able to get at least 7 hours of sleep (ideally 8) each night.

In addition, from now on, make it a habit to go to sleep at the same time each night. By doing so, you will program your body to recognize that it is time for it to prepare for sleep and the restoration that comes with it.

your sleep. Experiment with all of them and then choose those that you find to be most effective and suitable for you. Once you discover what works for you, continue to make use of it. Your goal is to make deep, restful sleep a nightly occurrence, something that occurs readily and easily for you.

Diet and Sleeping-Promoting Foods and Beverages

One of the primary ways you can improve your sleep is by following the dietary recommendations we shared in Chapter 4, focusing on meals that primarily contain alkalizing foods, instead of foods that create a buildup of acidic residues in your body. Doing so makes it easier for your body to perform its many health functions and, over time, can help release stored tensions in your body, making restful sleep easier to come by.

One of the keys to a restful night's sleep is to calm your brain. Certain foods contribute to restful sleep because they are rich in tryptophan. Tryptophan is an amino acid that the body uses to make serotonin, the neurotransmitter that slows down nerve signals so that your brain is able to relax. Tryptophan is also a precursor of melatonin. Although it is not advisable to have a full meal within a few hours of your bedtime, having a light snack of tryptophan-rich foods is permissible.

Turkey is a food that is rich in tryptophan (which explains why so many people feel ready for a nap soon after they finish their Thanksgiving meal). A small turkey sandwich eaten an hour or more before you go to bed, along with a cup of herbal tea, can be a delicious way to prepare for a good night's sleep.

Other tryptophan-rich foods include chicken, chickpeas, eggs, fish, lentils, milk, and yogurt. Certain needs and seeds, such as almonds, hazelnuts, pumpkin seeds, sesame seeds, and sunflower seeds also contain tryptophan and can therefore boost serotonin levels and enhance sleep when snacked on before bed. Just be sure not to overdo your snacking.

Another way to improve sleep has been recommended by practitioners of yoga for centuries. Pour a cup of milk into a pan and warm it just before it starts to boil. Then pour the milk into a cup and add a teaspoon of raw honey. Let the mixture cool for a few minutes, and then sip it slowly a few minutes before bedtime. This remedy has a very calming effect.

■ **NOTE:** If you are lactose intolerant, you can substitute almond milk for regular milk and still get the same benefits. Any of these snacks can help ready your brain, and therefore your body, for sleep. Choose whichever ones most appeal you.

Various herbal teas are also well-known for their ability to promote restful sleep. They include chamomile, hops, lemon balm, passionflower, skullcap, and valerian root, all of which can be prepared as teas.

Chamomile. Chamomile tea has long been used throughout Europe and Latin America to promote calmness and reduce tension. Its calming effects make it an excellent tea to drink in the evening to counteract tension before sleep. Chamomile is also an excellent digestive aid, and is therefore helpful for preventing sleep disturbances caused by indigestion.

Hops. Best known as an essential ingredient in beer, hops also has strong calming and sleep-promoting properties. In Germany and other European countries hops is licensed for use as a remedy for sleeping disorders, as well as for anxiety and tension. Taken as a tea before bedtime, hops, like chamomile, can be helpful for calming the mind, leading to a state of restfulness from which sleep can quickly follow.

Lemon balm. Lemon balm is an herb of the mint family that has been used by traditional herbalists for centuries as a remedy for insomnia. Its calming effects are also helpful for relieving anxiety, tension, and nervous disorders. A cup of lemon balm tea in the evening is therefore very conducive for a good night's sleep.

Passionflower. Passionflower is a natural sedative and is approved in Germany as an over-the-counter drug for treating nervous unrest. Passionflower can also enhance feelings of well-being because of its ability to promote calm. It is also effective as an aid for preventing and reversing high blood pressure. It can be used as a tea, or taken as an extract or tincture.

Skullcap. Skullcap is also a member of the mint family and is used traditionally as a nerve tonic and sedative. Skullcap also acts as a natural antispasmodic, making it an excellent choice for relieving muscle tension. It too can be taken as a tea, extract, or tincture.

Valerian root. Valerian root is perhaps the most commonly used herb for promoting sleep. It has been used for this purpose throughout Europe for centuries and is recognized as a natural tranquilizer. In Germany, valerian root in the form of tea and tinctures is approved as an over-the-counter sleep aid and as a remedy for states of anxiety and nervous excitation. Additionally, valerian root has been shown to promote warmth through the body, making it effective for relieving muscle pain. (Topical solutions of valerian root are now available for this purpose.) Valerian root is best taken as an extract 30 to 45 minutes before bedtime, at a dose of between 150 to 300 mg standardized to 0.5 percent of essential oil.

The above herbs can also be used in combination to further enhance their sleep-promoting qualities. A combination of chamomile, hops, and lemon balm is particularly delicious.

Sleep-Enchancing Nutritional Supplements

A variety of nutrients are known to improve and restore sleep. These include B vitamins, vitamin E, magnesium, and an amino acid known as GABA.

B Vitamins. Perhaps the most important vitamins for healthy sleep are those found in the vitamin B family. The B vitamins (collectively known as B-complex) play many important roles in your body, including supporting the health of your brain, eyes, intestines, liver, muscle, and skin. Additionally, B vitamins are essential for proper energy production and metabolism, and play an essential role in sleep because of the sedative effect they have on the nerves and their ability to help the human body cope with stress.

Specific B vitamins that have been shown to enhance sleep. B vitamins such as B3, B5, and B6 play an important role in helping your body get the sleep that is revitalizing.

Vitamin B3 (niacin). B3 helps to prolong REM (dream) sleep and prevent awakening during the night. It aids in normalizing sleep patterns. During the REM period your brain is active and dreaming although your body is inactive. This stage of sleep recharges your body and helps you stay focused during the day.

Dosage: It is suggested that you take 25 to 50 mg a day.

Vitamin B5 (pantothenic acid). B5 supports the adrenal glands and helps regulate hormone production. A deficiency of this B vitamin may result in sleep disorders and feelings of fatigue. In addition, B5 play a role in counteracting stress and anxiety, an important factor in sleep difficulties.

Dosage: It is suggested that you take 10 to 30 mg a day.

Vitamin B6 (Pyridoxine). B6 improves nerve function and is essential for serotonin production. A deficiency in serotonin may result in disrupted sleep patterns or the inability to get enough sleep.

Dosage: It is suggested that you take 50 to 100 mg once per day, either morning or evening.

Individual B vitamins are best taken with a complete B-complex formula to enhance their benefits. They can be taken at any time during the day or night.

Vitamin E. This is another vitamin that can aid in healthy sleep. It has also been shown to be effective for treating restless leg syndrome. When purchasing vitamin E, be sure to look for brands containing the natural, not the synthetic form. Synthetic forms are listed as DL-tocopherols, while natural forms are listed as D-tocopherols. Vitamin E is a fat-soluble vitamin, meaning that it is stored in fat cells.

Dosage: Can be unsafe at levels above 400 to 800 IUs taken once per day.

Magnesium. Among its literally hundreds of roles in the body, magnesium helps to nourish the nervous system and acts as a natural sedative and relaxant. It is also involved in the production of melatonin, a hormone that is essential for healthy sleep. Without enough magnesium your body is unable to produce and regulate melatonin, as well as other sleep-related hormones, that allow it to carry it out its natural sleep cycle.

Various studies have verified magnesium's ability to improve sleep via a variety of mechanisms. In addition to those mentioned above, magnesium regulates brain wave patterns and improves such patterns that are associated with insomnia. It also reduces levels of chronic, low-grade inflammation in the body, another marker linked to poor sleep. In addition, magnesium has been shown to reduce symptoms of restless leg syndrome and sleep apnea.

Improving Sleep With Melatonin

Melatonin is a hormone that is associated with healthy sleep. It is secreted by your brain's pineal gland, with the highest levels of production occurring during sleep. Healthy sleepers produce adequate amounts of melatonin each night, while people who struggle to get a good night's sleep typically do not. For this reason, a growing number of physicians recommend melatonin supplementation on a temporary basis when sleep proves difficult to come by. Melatonin has also been shown to increase deep sleep, REM (dream) sleep, and overall sleep efficiency, without producing any of the common "hangover" or stupor side effects common with both over-the-counter and prescription sleeping pills.

Melatonin supplements have been found to provide a host of health benefits, including boosting immune function, preventing premature aging, and helping to reverse a variety of sleep problems, including insomnia, the inability to stay asleep during the night, jet lag, and sleep problems caused by late shift work. In addition, numerous studies have found that melatonin supplements are completely non-toxic and therefore very safe for short-term use. (Even so, whenever you decide to use supplementation of any kind, be sure to inform your physician.)

Melatonin is available as an oral supplement in most health food stores around the country. Since it can promote sleep in as little as 30 minutes after it is consumed, you should only take melatonin at night, just before your bedtime. In addition, when you begin to use melatonin, your initial dose should be small—no more than one-half to one milligram (mg). (Most melatonin supplements come in a dose of between 1 to 3 mg per tablet. Buy the 1 mg tablets and cut them in half when you begin.)

If you find you need to increase your dose, do so in small increments (no more than an additional one milligram, and no higher than 3 mg per night). Once you start to realize the benefits of melatonin, it is also advisable that you stop using it for at least two weeks, so that your body doesn't stop producing its own amounts of melatonin. Then, if you still have trouble sleeping, you can start another cycle for another 2 to 4 weeks, ideally under your doctor's supervision.

Note: Since melatonin can enhance REM (dream) sleep, don't be alarmed if you experience vivid dreams when you begin using melatonin. Such dreams will subside over time once your body adjusts to your melatonin supplementation.

Before starting a melatonin supplementation program, consider some steps you can take to boost your body's own production of melatonin.

- Be sure to sleep in absolute darkness. That's because production of melatonin by the body best occurs in an environment of complete darkness.

- Unplug any electrical devices that may emit light while you sleep, including digital alarm clocks.

- Be sure that your curtains are completely drawn.

- For best results, consider sleeping with a sleep mask to prevent light from getting into your eyes.

- Additionally, if you find yourself awaking during the night to use the bathroom, get out of bed without turning on the lights if at all possible.

Dosage: For best results, take 400 to 500 mg of magnesium in the form of citrate, glycinate, or taurate 45 minutes before bedtime.

Gamma-aminobutyric acid (GABA). GABA is an amino acid. It acts as a major neurotransmitter and is widely distributed throughout your body's central nervous system (CNS). It is the most important and widespread inhibitory neurotransmitter in the brain, helping to prevent over-firing of nerve cells and decreasing overall neuron activities in the CNS. Over-firing can cause restlessness, spasmodic movements, irritability and anxiety. GABA is also utilized by the brain to create tranquility and calmness through the brain's metabolic processes, supporting a relaxed state of mind, and therefore promoting healthy sleep when taken before bedtime.

You can find GABA at your local health food store. All of the these nutrients are perfectly safe if taken within the suggested dosage ranges provided. If you aren't experiencing the level of sleep you desire, try supplementing with them for a few weeks to see if they make a difference for you.

Dosage: A typical dosage ranges from 125 to 500 mg. Start at the lower level and work up to the higher level if necessary.

Homeopathic Remedies

Homeopathy is a system of medicine that is used by approximately one billion people around the world, including the Royal Family of England, yet it remains virtually unknown by most people in the United States. Homeopathy was developed in the early 1800s by German physician Samuel Hahnemann. It is based on the principle that "like cures like," meaning that the same substance that in large doses produces the symptoms of an illness or health disorder is able to cure it in small doses.

Homeopathic remedies are perfectly safe. For best results, we suggest that you work with someone who is a classically trained homeopath (classical homeopathy refers to homeopathy as it was intended to be practiced by Dr. Hahnemann; in classical homeopathy, remedies are matched to the person, not the symptom). However, the following homeopathic remedies all lend themselves to self-care and can be very helpful for achieving better sleep; especially for acute sleeping problems (chronic sleep problems may require the assistance of a trained, classical homeopath).

Aconite. For sleep problems that are accompanied by restlessness and/or nightmares, or which are made worse after times of emotional shock or panic.

Arsenicum album. For problems that cause you to wake up between midnight and 2 AM feeling restless and apprehensive and/or accompanied by dreams of danger or disaster.

Belladonna. For people who have trouble sleeping due to being overly sensitive to external stimuli and/or who are angry, overly excited, or unable to easily fall asleep.

Chamomilla. For when you are unable to sleep because you feel wide awake and irritable.

Coculus. For when you feel too giddy or for when you are too tired to fall asleep.

Coffea. For when you experience sleep problems caused by a racing mind.

Ignatia. For insomnia accompanied by frequent yawns, and/or caused by emotional upset, and for sleep accompanied by nightmares.

Lycopodium. For people with overactive minds who are unable to let go of the day's affairs, and/or people who are heavy dreamers who awaken each time their dreams end.

Muriaticum acidum. For insomnia caused by grief; for extreme emotional sensitivity, and/or intolerance to sunlight.

Natrum muriaticum. For sleep problems caused by anxiety, upsetting dreams, and/or illness caused by emotional upset, and for people who are bothered by heat and sudden noise.

Nux vomica. For sleep problems to due to mental strain, overeating, alcohol consumption, withdrawal from alcohol or sleeping pills. For people who awaken in the middle of the night and then are unable to fall back asleep until around the time that they need to get up to start their day; this remedy is also useful for people who suffer from nightmares that leave them feeling irritable during the day.

Pulsatilla. For sleep problems that are characterized by first feeling too hot and then too cold, leaving you feeling restless; also useful for sleep problems caused by nightmares following a meal of rich food.

Rhus toxicodendron. For when you experience sleep problems accompanied by feelings of discomfort or pain, restlessness, and irritability, as well as a need to pace about.

For best results, take the above remedies in a dose of 30C approximately one hour before you go to bed. (You can find homeopathic remedies at most health food stores.) To find out more about homeopathy, contact The National Center for Homeopathy at www.homeopathic.org.

Aromatherapy

Aromatherapy is an ancient art which has been used for centuries by many different cultures. Over the last century the modern practice of aromatherapy has developed into a complete system of medicine that is widely used throughout Europe and is increasingly becoming popular in the US.

Aromatherapy uses the essential oils extracted from plants and herbs. Through various processes of distillation, the essences of plant flowers, leaves, branches, or root are distilled down into essential oils. These essential oils can be used in several different ways—added to bath water or a foot bath, added to a neutral 'carrier oil' (such as almond oil) to be diffused into the air, or in a massage, or inhaled. Whichever way the oils are used, they stimulate your sense of smell and, as the essential oils are absorbed into your bloodstream, they affect the limbic system (in your brain), which controls your emotions, moods and memory.

The benefits of aromatherapy are many, and have been verified by scientific research. Among the most common benefits are:

- enhanced immunity and greater resistance to infectious disease

- improved circulation

- improved digestion

- improved energy
- improved hormone function
- mood enhancement
- pain relief
- relief of muscle tension and spasms

Many aromatherapy oils are also excellent for stress relief, relaxation, and improved sleep.

There are three methods of application of essential oils that are most conducive for promoting relaxation and improved sleep.

1. **Inhalation:** This method is the very basis of aromatherapy, and the benefits of essential oils can be clearly seen when you use it. It's the simplest and most versatile aromatherapy technique, and there are several options for using it, such as an aromatherapy diffuser, candles, steam inhalation, a vaporizer, spray bottles, and more. (You can find diffusers and essential oils at most health food stores.) We suggest working with either a diffuser or a spray bottle.

- For the diffuser method, place the diffuser in your bedroom and add one or more of the following essential oils, being sure to follow the directions that come with the diffuser: chamomile, citronella, eucalyptus, or lavender. Then turn on the diffuser and let it run as you go to sleep.

- For spraying, be sure to use a glass spray bottle (4-ounce size is best). Fill the bottle with pure, filtered water, and then add 5 to 10 drops of lavender oil. Spray this solution about your room before you go to sleep. You can spray it lightly on your pillow.

2. **Taking an aromatherapy bath:** Adding essential oils to your bath is a very simple way to enjoy the effects of aromatherapy. At the end of a long day, enjoying the relaxing properties of bergamot, chamomile, lavender, or sandalwood essential oils added to a tub hot water can be a wonderfully soothing way to unwind and get ready for sleep.

Take a Bath for Better Sleep

Surely you know how relaxing a nice hot bath can be. But did you know that a bath before bedtime can significantly improve the quality of your sleep? It's true—a hot bath isn't just relaxing; it's also a powerful sleep aid.

This fact was conclusively shown to be true in a survey conducted in 1999 by the National Sleep Foundation. The survey found that respondents who took a hot bath before going to bed overwhelmingly reported that they fell asleep more quickly and easily and slept better than usual.

Other studies have found that taking a hot bath before bedtime can raise core body temperature approximately 2 degrees F, and that hot baths at night also increase the production of melatonin, the most important hormone necessary for healthy sleep. This increase in melatonin production was found to be caused as a natural reaction of the brain's pineal gland to increased body temperature caused by hot baths. The end result is a state of enhanced relaxation that carries over into better and deeper sleep.

You can add certain herbs to your bath to get even more sleep-enhancing benefits. To do so combine 1 to 2 tablespoons each of loose, dry chamomile, hops, lavender, and/or linden flowers. (These herbs are available from many health food stores, or via the Internet; Google "bulk herbs" to find sources.) Place the mixture in a muslin bag. Tie the bag closed and then place it in your bathtub as it fills with hot water. Keep the bag in the tub as you soak in it for 20 minutes. Not only will this herbal bath promote relaxation, it will also help to ease any muscle tension you may have. For even better results, have a cup of chamomile tea while you are soaking.

Here is an alternative method you can also try. Instead of using herbs, pour two cups of Epsom salts into your bath as it fills with hot water. Then soak in the solution for 20 minutes. Epsom salts contain a high amount of magnesium, a mineral that has potent relaxant properties. As you soak in the hot water, the magnesium contained in the salts will be absorbed into your body through your skin.

• Add 4 to 6 drops of your chosen oil to your bathwater, agitate well to mix, and then relax in the tub for 20 minutes. You can add more than one drop of oil, but don't exceed 8 drops of oil total.

• A footbath is a quick alternative to a soak in the tub. Use 3 to 4 drops maximum in this application.

3. **Massage:** This method involves the absorption of the essential oils through your skin, and is a wonderful way to achieve relaxing sleep for both you and your partner. The added therapeutic benefits of massage make for a relaxing bonus.

• It's important never to use undiluted ('neat') essential oils directly on your skin. You need to blend them with a carrier oil first. Aromatherapy oils are too strong to be applied directly to your skin, so they need to be blended with milder oils such as almond, avocado, jojoba, or sunflower. Many of the common carrier oils are nut-based, so if you're worried about the possibility of nut allergies, try sunflower or grape-seed oil instead.

• Although the essential oils are generally considered the 'important or active' part of the aromatherapy treatment, the carrier oils have their own special properties and benefits too. They contain vitamins and minerals, and are excellent moisturizing agents.

• To make an aromatherapy massage oil, add 5 drops of the essential oil of your choice (we recommend you try geranium, German or Roman chamomile, lavender, melissa, rosemary verbenone, or ylang-ylang) with 10 ml of a carrier oil, and shake well to blend.

• If you live alone, you can still get many of the benefits of aromatherapy massage simply by rubbing any of the above essential oils on your wrists, solar plexus, and temples before you retire for the night.

Acupressure

Acupressure is based on the same approach to health as acupuncture. The chief difference is that, instead of needles, acupressure is administered by using finger and thumb pressure on what traditional Chinese medicine refers to as *acupoints*, which are specific areas along the body's energetic pathways (meridians) that can both stimulate and calm the flow of energy (depending on what is needed) when pressure is applied to them. A significant benefit of acupressure, compared to acupuncture, is that it is an excellent form of self-care that anyone can learn how to do.

What follows are four acupuncture techniques you can do before bedtime in order to improve the quality of your sleep. Before you do them, take a bath or shower so that your hands and body are clean.

1. **Massage your ears:** According to acupuncture theory, the acu-points that run along the length of the outer ear correspond to all of the organs and energy pathways of the human body. Therefore, by massaging your ears, you can improve the functioning of all of your organ systems, bringing them into a state of balance or harmony. Do this exercise first before moving on to the other three techniques.

First, starting at your earlobes, use your thumbs and forefingers to simultaneously rub both of your ears, moving slowly up from your earlobes all the way up and then down to where your outer earlobes end, midway in the front of your ears. Once you complete this massage, repeat the process two more times, each time going more slowly and paying attention to areas along your outer ears that may be particular sore.

When you find sore spots, spend a few moments pressing into them, making sure that as you do so you are sitting comfortably and breathing fully in and out through your belly. Use firm, steady pressure. You will notice as you do this that the soreness starts to subside. When it does, move onto the next sore spot and continue this process until all areas of soreness in your ears have improved. Now you are ready to move on to the next acupressure point.

2. **Massage your feet: step 1:** Find the fleshy space on top of your foot, between your big and second toes. Feel for the sorest spot within this area and massage or press firmly into it for one minute, as you continue to breathe deeply and fully. Repeat this process twice more, then do the same thing with your other foot.

3. **Massage your feet: step 2:** When you are done with the second exercise, move up the top of your foot to the inside of your ankle. Feel for the fleshy part of your foot that is located between the front of your ankle and the bony prominence of your foot. Find where this area is sorest and press firmly into it for one minute. Repeat two more times, and then do the same thing for your other foot.

4. **Massage your brow:** After you have completed the three exercises above, turn off the lights and lie down in bed. Close your eyes and place your forefingers side by side just above the area where your eyebrows meet. Applying firm yet gentle pressure, move your fingers away from each other, sliding them along your brow, all the way to your temples. Do this slowly and in a relaxed manner. Then repeat this process four more times. This particular exercise helps to facilitate a shift from your normal waking brainwave (beta) patterns, to a calmer, more relaxed alpha state that is very conducive for falling asleep in a calm, relaxed manner.

Practice each of these acupressure techniques each night just before going to bed for at least the next two weeks and notice what happens.

Autogenic Training

Autogenic training is a relaxation technique that was developed in the early 1930s by Johannes Schultz, a German psychiatrist. The technique involves the daily practice of sessions that last around 15 minutes, usually in the morning, at lunch time, and in the evening. During each session, you will repeat a set of visualizations that induce a state of relaxation. Each session can be practiced while sitting comfortably or lying down.

Autogenic training is used by many physicians around the world to help their patients relieve stress and stress-induced disorders. It works by restoring the balance between the activity of the sympathetic ("flight or fight" response) and the parasympathetic ("rest and assimilate" response) branches of the autonomic nervous system. Studies have shown that autogenic training provides important health benefits, since the parasympathetic activity promotes better digestion and elimination, lowers blood pressure, slows heart rate, and enhances immune function. Because of its ability to relieve stress and promote physical relaxation, autogenic training is also highly effective as a sleep aid.

To perform autogenic training on yourself, sit comfortably in a chair or lie down. Close your eyes and mentally scan your body, noticing any areas of tension. Then mentally repeat to yourself the following suggestions:

My right arm is heavy.

My arms and legs are heavy and warm (repeat 3 times).

My heartbeat is calm and regular (repeat 3 times).

My solar plexus is warm (repeat 3 times).

My forehead is cool.

My neck and shoulders are heavy (repeat 3 times).

I am at peace (repeat 3 times).

My arms and legs are heavy and warm (repeat 3 times).

My heartbeat is calm and regular (repeat 3 times).

My solar plexus is warm (repeat 3 times).

My forehead is cool.

My neck and shoulders are heavy (repeat 3 times).

I am at peace (repeat 3 times).

My arms and legs are heavy and warm (repeat 3 times).

My heartbeat is calm and regular (repeat 3 times).

My solar plexus is warm (repeat 3 times).

My forehead is cool.

My neck and shoulders are heavy (repeat 3 times).

I am at peace (repeat 3 times).

Now count to ten, breathing deeply and easily and open your eyes when you are ready.

Try to take at least 10 minutes to perform this exercise, rather than rushing through it. Spend a few moments with each suggestion, feeling it occurring in your body. For best results, repeat this exercise three times a day, once in the morning, once in the afternoon, and once at night as you go to bed.

If you like, you can also record these suggestions. That way you can play the tape to yourself rather than having to remember

Improving Sleep By Getting More Sunshine In Your Life

Here's a very simple way to improve the quality of your sleep: Get out in the sun. Researchers have established a definite relationship between sunlight exposure during the day and restful sleep at night. This is due to the interaction of sunlight with the brain's pineal gland, which is responsible for producing the sleep hormone melatonin. Several studies have shown that melatonin production significantly drops, and in some cases can be completely inhibited, as a result of inadequate exposure to natural sunlight during the day.

Unfortunately, as a nation, too few of us get enough sunlight on a daily basis due to how much of our lives are spent indoors. Because of this, researchers have found that the average American is exposed to light levels of less than 100 lux (a measurement of light intensity) per day. This is the equivalent of the amount of light that would enter your eyes if you looked at a 100-watt light bulb from a distance of five feet in an otherwise dark room. By contrast, spending as little as ten minutes outside during a bright sunny day can expose you to up to 100,000 lux. And even on overcast, stormy days, outdoor light rarely dips below 500 lux.

Additional research has found that nighttime melatonin pro-

each of the suggestions and their proper sequence. However, for best results, we recommend that you eventually memorize the sequence of suggestions so that you can practice autogenic training any time that you may need to banish stress, and while you are in bed preparing to sleep.

Hand Warming

Hand warming is a self-care form of biofeedback. It is very easy to learn, and, once mastered, it can provide you with a key to your body's autonomic nervous system (ANS). The reason for that is

duction is directly related to the amount of serotonin production formed during the day. Serotonin is sometimes referred to as the "feel good" hormone because of the sense of calm it produces in the body. (People who are chronically depressed usually suffer from depleted levels of serotonin.) Multiple studies have shown that people who spend most of their time indoors have lower levels of serotonin compared to people who regularly spend a bit of time outdoors. Less serotonin production during the day means less melatonin production at night, and therefore poorer quality sleep.

You can avoid this problem simply by making it a point to spend as little as ten minutes outdoors each day. Ideally, you should do so during the morning during the hours of 7 to 9 AM, as sunlight exposure during this time will trigger greater production of serotonin for the rest of the day, leading to greater nighttime melatonin production. Research has also shown that exposure to sunlight between 7 to 9 helps to maintain proper function of your body's circadian rhythms and biological clock. Finally, sunlight exposure helps your body to produce and maintain adequate levels of vitamin D. So, if you want to sleep better and improve your overall health, try to make daily sunlight exposure part of your overall *Acid-Alkaline Lifestyle.*

because, in the nerve supply of the body from the sympathetic and the parasympathetic sides of the ANS, only the blood vessels in the hands and the feet have nerve supply controlled solely from the sympathetic side. When people warm their hands in this fashion, the only way they can do it is by lowering the sympathetic side of ANS activity. The parasympathetic isn't involved in hand warming, whereas heart rate, the hair rising up on your skin, the dilation of pupils, digestive track activity—all the autonomic organs, glands, and their functions are regulated by nerves that are controlled from both the parasympathetic and sympathetic. They have a "gas pedal" and a "break pedal", if you will, in much the same way that cars do.

The gas pedal revs the engine up and provides the energy to make the car go, and the brakes slow the car down or bring it to a stop. When we are under stress, it is like revving the engine and holding the brakes down at the same time. If we work under stress for a prolonged period, it's like driving the car with both the gas and the brake pedal pressed to the floor.

Hand warming is a method of self-regulation that is similar to lifting up on the accelerator in the car, without having to use the brakes. It eases up on the sympathetic outflow, restoring normal blood flow to the glands and organs. The heart slows down, breathing relaxes and deepens, and the body moves in a direction opposite to the fight or flight response. It leads to what Dr. Herbert Benson termed "the relaxation response." People feel it very definitely occurring at a certain point, when hand warmth is achieved. And, because of the deep relaxation and body warmth it provides, it can also help you to sleep better.

- Hold your hands in front of you with your palms toward you, and then bend your fingers gently forward until they are over the base of the hand, so that you form a kind of a hollow with your fingers and your palm. Then turn one hand over and slip its fingers into that space so that you're holding hands with yourself in a gentle way. Don't grip your fingers Then drop your hands into your lap, find a position that's comfortable, and let your shoulders, arms, and everything else relax. And then focus your attention just on your hands, feeling what they feel like, however they feel.

- Now see if you can feel your little fingers, their entire volume. Feel the proximal knuckle, then the distal knuckle, and then the tips of the little finger. Feel under the fingernail, the whole fingernail bed—just be aware of it in a sensory way. Most people can pretty quickly feel a tingling, a pulse, or a sensation of warmth as they focus on each finger. If you have a little temperature meter or thermometer taped to the end of your fingers, you will see that the temperature climbs. The goal is, while keeping your hands together, to get your temperature to 97 degrees or above. That's about where the relaxation response occurs. For some people, it occurs at a bit lower temperature. With practice, this becomes very easy to do and occurs automatically, like what happens when you focus sensory attention on your saliva glands.

For general relaxation, spend ten or fifteen minutes at a time practicing hand warming. For general stress management and to boost immune function, do it several times during the day. Because of its warming effect, we recommend that you practice hand warming just before you go to bed, since slightly increased body warmth is very conducive for a good night's sleep.

CONCLUSION

We cannot overemphasize how vitally important adequate levels of deep, restful sleep is to your overall health. In many ways, it may very well be the most vital component of *the Acid-Alkaline Lifestyle,* perhaps even more so than a healthy diet, because without quality sleep your body's numerous health function, including digesting the foods you eat and assimilating their nutrients, simply cannot occur at optimum levels due to the stressors that chronic poor sleep cause.

If you follow the guidelines we have shared in this chapter, and practice the self-care steps that we recommend, you should find the quality of your sleep improving within a few weeks to a month. If, after that time, you continue to experience sleep problems, we strongly advise that you speak with your doctor and/or seek out the assistance of a sleep specialist in your area. Failing to do so not only negatively impact your health, it can be outright dangerous.

Hopefully what you have learned in this chapter can help you achieve the quality of sleep that your desire. Pleasant dreams!

Conclusion

I t has been said that information is power. That is very true, *but only if that information is applied.* Now that you have read this book, you have the information you need to truly improve your health and the health of your loved ones. In order to do so, you must apply what you learn and be persistent.

Changes in health do not occur overnight, anymore than chronic health problems do. Both health and disease are the end result of accumulating factors that take root and then progress over time. Recognizing this fact, the ancient healers who created one of the world's oldest and most comprehensive healing systems—traditional Chinese medicine, or TCM—counseled that, for every year that a person had suffered with a chronic disease, one month of healing was necessary. Our hope, now that you have learned all that we have shared with you in these pages, is that you prove that maxim for yourself.

You may not yet appreciate it, but by reading this book you have given yourself a wide variety of healing tools and techniques that you can now use to first rebuild your health, and then to maintain it at levels you perhaps have never experienced before. Not only do you now understand how and why proper acid-alkaline balance is so vital to your overall health and well-being—a principle that is unknown or ignored by most physicians in our nation today—more importantly, you now have the knowledge you need to greatly enhance your body in keeping that pH balance intact, starting with your diet, and then by incorporating the rest of the elements of the Acid Alkaline Lifestyle into your daily routine. This knowledge will empower you to be able to actively take charge of your health simply because of the choices you make each day. The key, again, is to *apply what you've learned* and to *do so consistently.*

In many respects, the principles that underlie the Acid Alkaline Lifestyle are based on common sense. After all, throughout your life have you not repeatedly heard that in order to be healthy you need to eat right, exercise, get enough sleep, and manage stress? Of course you have. All doctors know this, as well, and most likely share that advice with all of their patients. In the vast majority of cases, however, that's as far as they go. Doctors today have neither the time, nor, in many cases, the awareness that you now possess thanks to reading this book, to properly educate their patients on *how* to effectively accomplish these goals, let alone explain the importance of acid-alkaline balance. How can they when the average time spent by patients with their doctors during office visits is now less than five minutes?

As a result, common sense, when it comes to today's health care system, is far from common. In fact, it's almost non-existent. The truth is that you cannot depend on your doctor to provide you with all of the information you require to be and stay healthy because they simply do not have the time to share it with you and, in many cases, are further disadvantaged by not knowing it themselves, given how extensively focused their medical training is on drug-based symptom care *after* their patients become sick. Such an emphasis has little to do with actual health and, as we mentioned in our Introduction, is one of the primary reasons why health care costs in America today are so exorbitantly expensive.

If you are like most people, then no doubt much of what we shared with you is new and unfamiliar information. Should that be the case, you may find yourself having doubts about it. If so, that's fine. We are not asking you to believe us. Rather, we hope that you will take it upon yourself to commit to implementing our suggestions to discover whether or not they actually have value for you. In fact, we encourage you to be skeptical at first.

Yet, at the same time, we also encourage you to allot enough time as you apply what you have learned in order to give the changes you will be making to your lifestyle enough time to produce results. In many cases, this means applying your newfound knowledge for at least 30 to 90 days. In other cases, it may take longer than that, possibly up to six months, or even a year, depending on a person's current state of health. If you make such a commitment, we are confident that you will begin to experience significant positive changes in your health, energy level, and the overall health status of your "body, mind, and Spirit."

Finally, we want you to know that we do not expect you to rigidly adhere to everything we have shared with you. From time to time, you may find yourself wanting to indulge in old habits— an acidifying hamburger and fries, for example, or a loss of sleep due to staying up late with friends. If that is the case, by all means do so and enjoy yourself. Over time, however, the more that you adopt the Acid-Alkaline Lifestyle, don't be surprised if you find that you want to engage in such indulgences less and less because of how good following our recommendations makes you feel.

Like everything else in life, your health is a journey complete with ups and downs. Therefore it is very important that you proceed at your own pace, being persistent and doing the best you can. As it's been said, "The journey of a thousand miles begins with the first step." You took that first step when you began reading this book, and took many other steps by reading it through to the end. Keep on walking by making use of what you have learned for new vistas of well-being are waiting in front of you.

To your health!

Glossary of Terms

acid. Any substance in the body that gives off hydrogen ions when it is dissolved in water. Such substances have a pH value of less than 7.0. (Also see *pH.*)

acid-alkaline balance. A necessary element of health in the body created by a balanced state of acidic and alkaline substances in the body's fluids and tissues.

acidifying. The effect caused by any substance that lowers pH values below 7.0.

acidosis. This condition is a state of chronic over-acidity in the body's tissues and fluids.

adenosine triphosphate. A fuel produced by the cells that is synthesized from oxygen and glucose. It is essential for powering the cells' sodium-potassium pumps, which deliver oxygen and vital nutrients to the cells and transport cellular waste.

aerobic. Literally means "with oxygen." A term used to designate any activity that introduces or increases oxygen supply.

aerobic exercise. Any form of exercise that increases the efficiency of oxygen intake by the lungs and hearts. Aerobic exercises include jogging, rebounding, running, swimming, tai chi, and yoga breathing techniques.

alkaline. Having a pH value greater than 7.0.

alkalis. Substances that can neutralize acids and that have a pH value greater than 7.0.

alkalizing. One produces an alkaline state and reduces acidity.

alkalosis. This is a state of excessive or over-alkalinity. Although rare, a state of chronic alkalosis can be life-threatening.

amino acid. These are any of 25 substances used by the body to synthesize proteins.

anaerobic. A term used to describe a condition of little to no oxygen. In the human body, an anaerobic state is ideal for the growth of harmful microorganisms such as bacteria, fungi, and viruses.

ANS. See *autonomic nervous system.*

antioxidant. Any substance that slows down or reverses the effects of oxidation in the body caused by cell-damaging free-radicals is considered to be an antioxidant. Antioxidant nutrients include vitamins A, C, and E, beta carotene, CoQ10, selenium, and zinc.

arrhythmia. An abnormal or irregular heartbeat.

arteriosclerosis. A hardening of the arteries caused by calcium and/or plaque buildup inside the walls of the arteries; also known as *atherosclerosis.*

ATP. See *adenosine triphosphate.*

autonomic nervous system. The part of the nervous system that is responsible for controlling and regulating the body's involuntary functions, such as breathing, circulation, and endocrine function. The autonomic nervous system consists of two parts: the sympathetic and the parasympathetic nervous systems.

bicarbonate. A form of acid salt secreted by the pancreas that neutralizes or buffers hydrochloric acid.

Candida albicans. A naturally occurring yeast fungus in the digestive tract which, when overgrown, can create a variety of disease symptoms and lead to candidiasis or systemic yeast infection.

Candidiasis. A chronic and systemic yeast infection caused by the overgrowth of the fungus *Candida albicans.* Also known simply as candida, candidiasis can result in a variety of disease conditions, including allergy, chronic fatigue syndrome, and impaired immunity.

carcinogens. Any substances, such as environmental toxins, that can cause cancerous changes in the body's cells and genes.

central nervous system. That part of the nervous system consisting of the brain, spinal cord, and major nerve chords that run along the length of the spine and through the vertebrae sending nerve impulses from the brain throughout the rest of the body.

CFS. See *chronic fatigue syndrome*.

Chronic fatigue syndrome. An illness characterized by severe and prolonged exhaustion. Because its cause is not specific, it is known as a syndrome rather than a disease (diseases are caused by known specific agents), and can often be accompanied by depression, headache, mental confusion, mild fever, muscle ache or weakness, and/or sore throat.

EFAs. See *essential fatty acids*.

electrolyte. This is any substance, in liquid form, which is capable of conducting an electric current through the body. Acids, bases, and salts are common forms of electrolytes. Electrolytes help regulate fluid levels in the body, maintain proper pH, and play a vital role in the transmission of nerve impulses from the brain to the rest of the body.

endocrine. This term pertains to any gland that produces one or more hormones.

endocrine system. This system of the body produces and regulates the secretion of hormones in the body. It consists of the following glands: hypothalamus, pituitary, thyroid/parathyroid, thymus, adrenal, pancreas, testes (in men), and ovaries (in women).

essential fatty acids. These fats are required by the body's cells to ensure proper cell function. Essential fatty acids cannot be manufactured by the body, and therefore must be supplied by the diet in order to ensure good health. There are two essential fatty acids: alpha linolenic acid of the omega-3 family and linoleic acid of the omega-6 family.

environmental illness. An illness caused by exposure to pollutants and toxins in the environment (air, water, and/or land). Such illnesses can include otherwise unexplained allergies, anxiety and depression, arrhythmia, behavioral problems, chronic fatigue syndrome, eczema and hives, edema, gastrointestinal disorders, headache, muscle ache, respiratory conditions, and sleep disorders.

environmental toxins. Chemicals and other substances released into the environment (air, land, and/or water) that are hazardous to human health due to how they negatively impact the body.

enzyme. Substances in the body and contained in certain foods (primarily fruits and vegetables) that act as catalysts for biochemical reactions. Enzymes are necessary for every single process that the body performs including breathing, digestion, immune function, reproduction, proper organ function, as well as speech, thought, and movement. A certain class of enzymes, known as food or digestive enzymes are available as nutritional supplements to assist in the digestion of carbohydrates, fats, fibers, and proteins.

free-radical. A molecule that is unstable and negatively charged that can cause premature aging and disease. Free-radicals naturally occur in the body during energy production, but they can also be created in unhealthy amounts by the buildup of toxins and waste products in the body, poor diet, nutritional deficiencies, and exposure to environmental toxins and radiation.

genetic predisposition. A term used to describe a person's predisposition to certain disease and illnesses based on hereditary factors passed down from generation to generation through the genes.

HCL. See *hydrochloric acid.*

heat shock protein. This is a type of protein required by the body to facilitate cellular repair. Heat shock proteins does help repair cells by aiding in the disposal of old or damaged proteins, while helping to build and transport new proteins.

homeostasis. A term used to describe the body's inherent self-regulating mechanisms, which seek always to maintain equilibrium or balance, within all of the body's systems.

hormone. A chemical produced by the endocrine glands and secreted into the bloodstream in order to help regulate proper cell and organ function, aid in the body's response to stress, and assist in proper metabolism and energy production in within the mitochondria.

hydrochloric acid. An acid secreted by the stomach to breakdown and help digest food.

hydrogen ion. A single, unstable proton created when hydrogen molecules are dissolved in water through a process known as *dissociation* (see above). All acids in the body give off hydrogen ions when they are dissolved in water. pH values are determined according to the concentration of hydrogen ions a substance has.

hydrogen ion concentration. The measurement used to determine a substance's pH value. The greater the concentration of hydrogen ions in a substance, the more acidic it is, while the substances with lesser concentrations are considered neutral or alkaline.

hyperglycemia. High blood sugar caused by an abnormally high concentration of sugar in the bloodstream.

hyperventilation. Extremely rapid or deep breathing that can result in dizziness and fainting due to the rapid loss of carbon dioxide during exhalation.

hypoglycemia. Low blood sugar caused by less than normal concentrations of sugar in the bloodstream.

inflammation. A condition caused by acid buildup that can occur anywhere in the body, leading to illnesses ending with "*-itis*," a suffix used to indicate an inflammatory condition. Inflammation of the joints can cause arth*ritis*, for example, while inflammation of the nerves can lead to neu*ritis*, inflammation in the lungs can cause bronc*hitis*. Inflammation of the gastrointestinal tract can result in col*itis* or enter*itis*. Another sign of inflammation in the body is burning pains in various other organs.

ion. An atom or group of atoms with an electrical charge caused when a neutral atom or group of atoms gains or losses one or more electrons during chemical reactions. When ions lose electrons they become positively charged, and when they gain electrons, they become negatively charged.

jaundice. This disease condition of the liver is characterized by abnormally yellowish coloration in the eyeballs, skin, and/or urine. Jaundice is caused by liver dysfunction that results in increased amounts of bile pigments entering and remaining in the bloodstream.

lactic acid. A waste product produced by the fermentation of sugar (glucose) by the cells. Lactic acid buildup increases acidity in the body, making it more difficult for healthy cells to obtain and efficiently make use of oxygen.

lymph. This is a clear, yellowish fluid that is part of the lymphatic system. Lymph transports vital nutrients to the cells and helps expel cellular toxins.

lymphatic system. The lymphatic system acts as the body's filtration system, helping to transport vital nutrients and other essential elements to the cells, while eliminating cellular wastes, an integral part of the immune system. When the lymphatic system becomes clogged or congested due to the buildup of acid wastes, cell function becomes diminished due to diminished nutrient supply and the increased buildup of intercellular wastes, setting the stage for disease to occur.

metabolism. A term used to describe the biochemical reactions and interactions within the body that result in the production of energy and nutrients necessary to sustain good health.

mind/body medicine. The area is a field of medicine that studies the interrelationships between thoughts, emotions, attitudes and beliefs and their ability to create health and disease. Common types of mind/body medicine include biofeedback therapy, cognitive therapy, guided imagery and visualization, hypnosis, and meditation.

mitochondria. The cells' internal energy factories, the mitochondria, produce energy using a fuel called adenosine triphosphate (see above), a substance synthesized from oxygen and glucose. The mitochondria also play an essential role in all intracellular enzyme activity.

mole. A term used to describe the molecular weight of a substance. pH is determined by measuring the concentration of hydrogen ions, which is calculated as moles per liter.

molecule. A molecule is the smallest quantity into which a substance can be reduced without losing any of its characteristics. The smallest molecular structures consist of a single atom, while a combination of two or more atoms create molecular chemical compounds.

molecular weight. See *mole.*

neuro-function. This term refers to the function of the nervous system.

neuromuscular. Of, relating to, or involving both the nerves and muscles.

neurotransmitter. Any biochemical substance that transmits or inhibits nerve impulses from nerve cells to other cells of the body.

over-alkalinity. A condition characterized by an excessively high alkaline pH. See also *alkalosis.*

over-breathing. See *hyperventilation.*

parasympathetic nervous system. The part of the autonomic nervous system responsible for conserving the body's energy supply. Physiological effects of the parasympathetic nervous system include constriction of the pupils, slowing of the heartbeat, and overall calming effects.

pathogen. Any form of microorganism, such as bacteria, fungi, or viruses, capable of causing disease.

peripheral nerves. Nerves located outside of the central nervous system. Peripheral nerves include all cranial nerves, all nerves along the spine and the spine's branches to the entire body, sensory nerves, and nervous of the parasympathetic and sympathetic nervous system.

pH. Literally means "potential for hydrogen," the term pH refers to a scale of measurement of the acidity or alkalinity of any substance, including body tissues and fluids. The pH scale runs from 0 to 14, with 7.0 considered neutral. pH values below 7.0 are considered acidic, and pH values above 7.0 are considered alkaline.

pH factor. This is the underlying factor that determines whether or not the body is in a state of acid-alkaline balance.

pH strip. A type of tape used to measure the pH of saliva or urine.

physiology. This term refers to the collective functions and processes of the body. Also refers to the branch of biology that deals with the body's functions and processes.

potential for hydrogen. This phrase is the literal meaning of the term pH (see *pH*).

Prostatitis. Usually caused by infection, this is an inflammation of the prostate gland.

psychosocial stress. Stress caused by relationship difficulties, social isolation, and a lack of social support.

psycho-spiritual stress. Stress caused as the result of a crisis of faith or values, questions about one's purpose in life, the lack of meaningful work, or the involvement of day to day activities that do not reflect one's core beliefs.

qigong. A form of exercise developed in China over two thousand years ago that is characterized by slow stretching movements accompanied by focused breathing and meditative concentration. (See also *Tai chi.*)

relaxation response. A term coined by Herbert Benson, M.D., of Harvard Medical School, to describe the physiological effects produced when the body enters a calm state of relaxation as a result of meditation or simply sitting still while focused on one's breathing.

serotonin. This hormone acts as a "feel good" neurotransmitter in the brain, and which influences sleep, mood, and brain functions related to sensory perception.

sodium-potassium levels. Levels showing the balance between sodium and potassium within and without the cell walls. Inside the cells, the potassium has to remain high and the sodium has to remain low for the body's energy, which is electrical in nature, to be generated. Outside the cell, the concentrations of sodium and potassium are reversed; potassium levels are low and sodium levels are high.

stressor. This term refers to an internal or external factor that can trigger stress. Internal stressors include harmful or inaccurate thoughts and beliefs, and suppressed and inappropriately expressed emotions. External stressors include unhealthy foods, environmental toxins, and pathogens.

subluxation. A condition characterized by a misalignment in of the spine or vertebrae.

sympathetic nervous system. The aspect of the autonomic nervous system that governs how the body expends energy. It consists of the primarily of the nerves that supply impulses to the body's involuntary muscles and is activated during times of stress. Physiological effects of the sympathetic nervous system include accelerated heart beat, increased blood pressure, and dilation of the pupils.

"syndrome condition." A term used to designate any disease condition that cannot be attributed to a specific cause. Common syndrome conditions include chronic fatigue syndrome, environmental illness, and fibromyalgia.

tai chi. A form of exercise developed in China over two thousand years ago that is characterized by slow stretching movements accompanied by focused breathing and meditative concentration.

tetany. A disorder that is characterized by muscle spasm and/or muscle cramps that can be quite painful. Tetany can often result from hyperventilation or over-breathing.

Venous Plasma pH Test. This test is the most accurate test for measuring the pH of the blood. It needs to be administered by a physician, who withdraws a vial of bottle from the vein in the arm and then sends the blood to a licensed laboratory for testing.

vertebrae. The bone segments that make up the spinal column.

yeast infection. A condition caused by the overgrowth of naturally occurring yeast in the intestinal tract, mouth, or vagina. The most common type of yeast infection is candidiasis, caused by the overgrowth of the yeast *Candida albicans*.

About the Authors

Larry Trivieri, Jr., is a nationally recognized authority on holistic, integrative, and non-drug-based healing methods, with more than 30 years of personal experience in exploring techniques for optimal wellness and human transformation, including acid-alkaline balance. During that time, Trivieri has interviewed and studied with more than 400 of the world's top physicians and other health practitioners in over 50 disciplines in the holistic health field.

Trivieri is the author or co-author of nearly 20 books on health, including *The Acid-Alkaline Food Guide, Juice Alive, The American Holistic Medical Association Guide to Holistic Health, The Self-Care Guide to Holistic Medicine,* and *Health on the Edge: Visionary Views of Healing in the New Millennium.* He also served as editor and principal writer of both editions of the landmark health encyclopedia, *Alternative Medicine: The Definitive Guide,* and has written over 200 articles for Internet-based health sites, including 1Healthy-World.com and IntegrativeHealthReview.com and its online journal *iThrive.* He has also written numerous feature articles for a variety of publications, including *Alternative Medicine,* for which he also served as contributing editor from 1999 through 2002; *Natural Health, Natural Solutions,* and *Yoga Journal.* He has also been written about in a number of national publications, including *The Washington Post.*

Trivieri is dedicated to sharing the wealth of potentially life-saving information he has learned about with as wide an audience as possible in order to help usher in a new era of wellness and health care in the twenty-first century. To that end, he also lectures about health nationwide, and has been a featured guest on numerous TV and radio shows across the United States.

Neil Raff, MD, is medical director at Advanced Medicine of Mount Kisco, P.C. He has specialized in Internal Medicine and Gastroenterology for over 30 years. He graduated from Johns Hopkins School of Medicine in 1961, and went on to complete his medical internship at NYU-Bellevue, and his medical residency and gastroenterology fellowship at Bronx VA Hospital. While serving in the United States Air Force (USAF) he became a member of the Academy of Psychosomatic Medicine, which integrates physical and psychological function (the mind-body connection). Dr. Raff is Certified Nutritional Specialist (C.N.S.) whose ever-expanding interest in complementary medicine has led him to combine his professional medical practices with natural and nutritional therapies. Dr. Raff has appeared on various health and wellness shows, Gary Null's radio show: Natural Living, and as a speaker at Gilda's Club.

With his training as an Internist and Gastroenterologist, Dr. Raff created Advanced Medicine of Mt. Kisco, in Mt. Kisco, NY, in order to integrate the best of medical traditions, emphasizing nutrition and supplements to treat each person's individual needs and deficiencies. His guiding mantra with his patients is *"Taking time to listen to the patient is the most important diagnostic test there is."* For more information about Dr. Raff, visit his website, www.neilraffmd.com.

Index

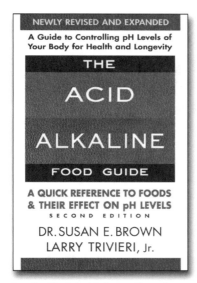
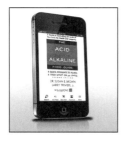

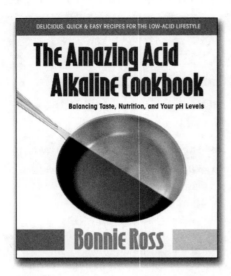

THE AMAZING ACID-ALKALINE COOKBOOK

Balancing Taste, Nutrition, and Your pH Levels

Bonnie Ross

It is no secret that the foods you eat have a direct impact on your health. But did you know that for optimum health, your body needs the proper balance of acid and alkaline compounds, which are influenced by diet? The problem is that, as a society, we tend to consume large amounts of sugar-laden, meat-based, and highly processed foods, all of which acidify the body. This, in turn, makes us prone to fatigue, arthritis, osteoporosis, as well as a number of more serious health conditions such as diabetes, cardiovascular disease, and kidney disease.

Fortunately, author Bonnie Ross has a solution with *The Amazing Acid-Alkaline Cookbook.* Divided into two parts, the book opens with the basics of the pH-balanced lifestyle, including an explanation of how an overly acidic body weakens the immune system and wreaks havoc on wellness. To help make your dietary choices easy, the author also provides a comprehensive reader-friendly chart that categorizes a wide variety of foods according to their acidifying or alkalizing qualities. Part Two contains over 140 kitchen-tested recipes for a vast array of perfectly balanced dishes that are both satisfying and delicious. Choose from a wonderful selection of taste-tempting breakfast favorites, soups, salads, snacks, and sides, as well as an impressive array of delectable main dishes. Also included are recipes for breads, biscuits, and other baked goods, plus a dessert chapter packed with sweet treats that are sure to please!

Good health is within your reach. *The Amazing Acid-Alkaline Cookbook* will show you just how easy it is to make flavorful meals that will naturally correct your body's pH balance, helping you regain or maintain vigor and well-being.

$17.95 US • 176 pages • 7.5 x 9-inch quality paperback• ISBN 978-0-7570-0316-5

IN BALANCE FOR LIFE

Understanding and Maximizing Your Body's pH Factor

Alex Guerrero

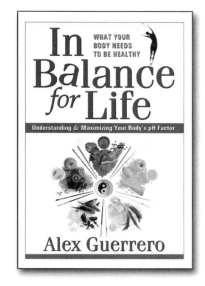

The principle of balance is not new. It forms the very foundation of both Eastern and Western philosophies, from Aristotle to Confucius. As it relates to health, it has been around just as long, from the development of traditional Chinese medicine to the treatments used by Hippocrates and Galen. What is new, however, is a scientifically based application that can improve numerous disorders and maximize your health.

Imagine that the human body has an internal mechanism that keeps two basic types of chemicals--acid and alkali--in balance. When your body becomes either too acidic or too alkaline, you become susceptible to a host of disorders. When balance is restored, however, so is your health. In this brilliant book, renowned health expert Alex Guerrero explains how you can become well--now and for an extended lifetime—by restoring your pH balance. The author first describes how you can assess your health. He then provides a plan, including a fourteen-day diet and a simple program of supplements, that will bring your body back into balance. You'll even find a selection of recipes that will tempt your taste buds as you reclaim your health and well-being.

In Balance for Life offers a revolutionary look at why we become ill. It also presents the simple steps you can follow—each and every day—to enjoy boundless vitality and optimal well-being.

$15.95 US • 192 pages • 6 x 9-inch quality paperback • ISBN 978-0-7570-0264-9

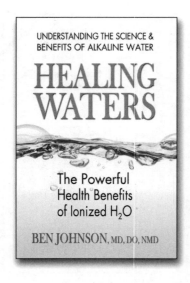

UNDERSTANDING THE SCIENCE &
BENEFITS OF ALKALINE WATER

HEALING WATERS

The Powerful
Health Benefits
of Ionized H₂O

BEN JOHNSON, MD, DO, NMD

HEALING WATERS

The Powerful Health Benefits of Ionized H2O

Ben Johnson, MD, DO, NMD

Acid-alkaline balance is the key to optimum health, and now you can achieve it simply by drinking nature's most bountiful liquid—water. In this revolutionary book, Dr. Ben Johnson guides you to oxygen-rich ionized water, H_2O that is altered through the safe and simple process of electrolysis. Filled with antioxidants and alkalizing minerals, ionized water not only provides the body with the substance that is essential to all functions, but also restores balance and maximizes well-being.

Healing Waters begins by explaining why water is crucial to good health. It then explores the importance of the body's acid-alkaline balance and examines why problems with this balance are responsible for many chronic conditions, such as diabetes and high blood pressure. Most important, the author reveals everything you need to know about ionized water, a natural remedy that is both pure and amazingly effective. You will learn how to buy, install, and use your own water ionizer so that your kitchen is turned into a healthful oasis. You will discover that even the byproducts of the ionizing process can be used as a tool to enhance well-being. The author even provides nutritional tips for balancing your body easily and naturally.

The Fountain of Youth may be just another legend, but with *Healing Waters,* you will understand that a good source of health and longevity may be no farther than your own home.

$15.95 US • 128 pages • 6 x 9-inch quality paperback • ISBN 978-0-7570-0328-8

**For more information about our books,
visit our website at www.squareonepublishers.com**